"*ForeverFitU* is a down-to-earth, practical, and playful call to action book. The stories of everyday folks will draw those in who need to know being ForeverFit really is a possibility in their lives. *ForeverFitU* is a fun, informative, encouraging tool in the pursuit of total well-being."

Kate Larsen
Executive coach and author of
Progress Not Perfection: Your Journey Matters

"Very seldom do I read books twice but this one I did. The time, effort, knowledge and precision Scott put into ForeverFitU is amazing. Being a Contestant on Season 9 of *The Biggest Loser* and reading these stories about how people made fitness a permanent part of their life was very inspiring to me. ForeverFitU has even helped me with my own continuing journey."

O'Neal Hampton, Jr.
Contestant on Season 9 of NBC's
The Biggest Loser

ForeverFitU

MAKING FITNESS A LIFESTYLE THAT LASTS A LIFETIME

SCOTT FJELSTED, CPT

BALBOA.
PRESS

A DIVISION OF HAY HOUSE

Balboa Press books may be ordered through booksellers or by contacting:

The views expressed in this work are solely those of the author and do not necessarily reflect the views of the publisher, and the publisher hereby disclaims any responsibility for them.

Balboa Press
A Division of Hay House
1663 Liberty Drive
Bloomington, IN 47403
www.balboapress.com
1-(877) 407-4847

Because of the dynamic nature of the Internet, any web addresses or links contained in this book may have changed since publication and may no longer be valid. The views expressed in this work are solely those of the author and do not necessarily reflect the views of the publisher, and the publisher hereby disclaims any responsibility for them.

The author of this book does not dispense medical advice or prescribe the use of any technique as a form of treatment for physical, emotional, or medical problems without the advice of a physician, either directly or indirectly. The intent of the author is only to offer information of a general nature to help you in your quest for emotional and spiritual well-being. In the event you use any of the information in this book for yourself, which is your constitutional right, the author and the publisher assume no responsibility for your actions.

Any people depicted in stock imagery provided by Thinkstock are models, and such images are being used for illustrative purposes only.
Certain stock imagery © Thinkstock.

Printed in the United States of America

ISBN 978-1-4525-3872-3 (sc)
ISBN 978-1-4525-3873-0 (hc)
ISBN 978-1-4525-3874-7 (ebk)

Library of Congress Control Number: 2011916279

Balboa Press rev. date: 10/05/2011

To our health, possibly the greatest gift given to us.

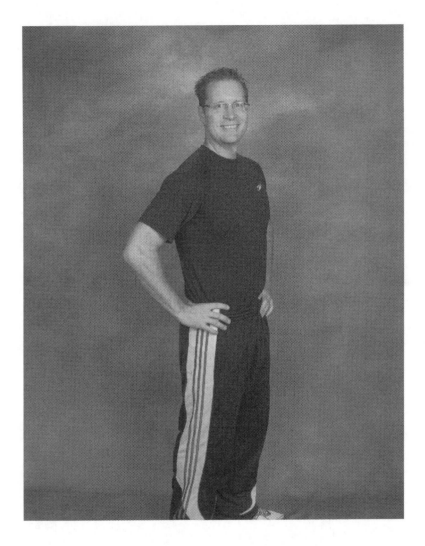

"Forever begins now."
Scott Fjelsted

Contents

Foreword

By O'Neal Hampton, Jr.
Contestant on Season 9 of NBC's *The Biggest Loser*

I first met Scott and his wife Meredith (he affectionately calls her Sunshine) on a plane ride to Arizona. Scott explained to me that he was a personal trainer and an author in the process of writing a book about making fitness a lifestyle that lasts a lifetime. We exchanged business cards. He said if I ever needed help at my fitness resort to give him a call. I thought, "yeah yeah", I will put his card with the stack from people I have at home. A few months passed before we actually met face to face again. That meeting told me a couple of things—our friendship was meant to be and so was this book. The one thing I could tell from the very beginning of our friendship is that he was a man with a strong faith in the Lord.

A month or so later I was in Los Angeles for knee surgery and had ForeverFitU to read. I could not believe what Scott had put to paper. Very seldom do I read books twice but this one I did. The time, effort, knowledge and precision Scott put into ForeverFitU is amazing. Being a Contestant on Season 9 of *The Biggest Loser* and reading these stories about how people made fitness a permanent part of their life was very inspiring to me. ForeverFitU has even helped me with my own continuing journey.

One of the biggest things I got from ForeverFitU is when you choose your behavior you choose your consequences.

Preface

Do you have a hard time sticking to an exercise routine? Have you made exercise a regular part of your life, perhaps for weeks to years, only to once again let it fall to the wayside? Do you work with a personal trainer but find it difficult to exercise on your own? Do you wonder why losing weight just doesn't motivate you enough to keep going? Do you feel you are on a last-ditch effort to make fitness a lasting lifestyle? Is this the first time in your life you are thinking about beginning an exercise program, and you are afraid of failure? If any or all of these are true for you, welcome to ForeverFitU.

This book is written with the intention of showing you how to make fitness a lifestyle that will last you a lifetime. Mother Theresa stated, "We cannot do great things in this world. We can only do little things with great love." I pray that ForeverFitU will be that little thing for you.

Having been a personal trainer since 1998, I have had thousands come to me to get set up on fitness regimens. After getting their initial fitness program, I noticed that more than 95 percent quit within a relatively short time. While these people were quitting at a rapid rate, about 5 percent of the people kept exercising consistently. I began to know them by name. For the rest of this book, I will refer to this group of people as "ForeverFit."

As the years went by, I became increasingly frustrated with the massive dropout rate of those who came to me. I came to realize that although I was giving them the proper exercises to do, I wasn't giving them any tools to help them make this new habit last. After investigation, I realized that there weren't any tools to directly address this problem.

One day, as I was working with one of my ForeverFit clients, I said, "I wonder what it is that all of you have that others who struggle with consistent exercise routines don't have. How do you keep exercise as a habit?" Since I knew that I didn't have all the answers, I began interviewing my closest ForeverFit friends and family. I asked them such questions as:

- How do you make time to exercise?
- What do you tell yourself on a daily basis to get yourself to exercise?
- Where is exercise on your priority list?
- What is the number one reason you exercise?
- How do you get yourself to exercise when you are unmotivated?

Getting these questions and others answered solved my first problem. The second problem was figuring out how to help people change their current mentalities to ForeverFit ones. Since I have been blessed with many great teachers along my path of personal growth and change, I now have tools that have helped me so I can help you. Problem solved. ForeverFitU was born.

I am a true believer in the idea that if you want what someone else has, you have to do what he or she did to get it, and then you will one day have it, too. Want to be wealthy? Learn from a self-made millionaire. Want a long, loving, lasting marriage? Learn from couples who have been happily married fifty-plus years. Want to learn to make exercise a permanent habit? Read and apply the principles in *ForeverFitU*.

You will hear stories of ForeverFit folks from different backgrounds, ages, and genders that have all become ForeverFit in different ways and time frames. Within this group are CEOs, business owners, an ex-police officer, a vice president of a large company, a former Miss Minnesota, my mom, accountants, an electrician, yoga instructors, personal trainers, fitness instructors, many computer/

desk workers, cancer survivors, nurses, teachers, sales people, mothers, fathers, grandmas, and grandpas. Some have had periods of extended breaks away from exercise due to illness, family issues, laziness, etc., but they all came back. They are all living the incredibly busy lives we all are, yet they never use time as an excuse to forego exercise. Their stories are there to help you see that your past has nothing to do with whether or not you will succeed. Whether you are old or young, are male or female, work sixty hours a week or are a stay-at-home parent, or are of any race, have any physical or mental issue—it doesn't have anything to do with your ability to become ForeverFit. If you can *move*, you can *improve!*

So, what makes someone qualify as a ForeverFit (FF) person? Although there are no specific parameters, ForeverFit people treat the habit of exercise like they do brushing their teeth. It is just something they do each day. You rarely hear them talking about it, and they rarely take time away from it. Fitness is ingrained in them. Some struggle for a long time before becoming ForeverFit, while others make it a habit from the first day. Regardless of their path, all of them have crossed over to becoming ForeverFit. It is that place where all who begin an exercise program strive to be. You are about to discover their secrets.

ACKNOWLEDGMENTS

How can I say "thank you" enough to all who have helped me with not only the information in ForeverFitU, but through the entire process that it has undergone to get it published? First, I have to thank God, for without divine intervention, this book would have never come to be. I thank God for putting the idea in my head, having it put to paper so easily, and for all of the wonderful individuals put in my path that have helped me so much on this publishing journey.

Thank you, Meredith, my wife and number one fan. Thank you for always believing in me and my vision to help people make fitness a lifestyle that lasts a lifetime. Thank you for loving me through everything in life. Thank you for being my up when I am down, and for being the best assistant anyone could dream of. I love you.

Thank you to Colin and Aidan, my two sons. I love you more than words can say, and you are a big reason I stay ForeverFit. I pray I am a positive influence in your lives, and I thank you for putting up with me in the moments I am not.

Thank you, Mom, for showing me through your actions that fitness can be as normal a part of life as brushing your teeth. You have influenced not only my exercise habits, but my faith as well.

Thank you to my family and all of my friends, coworkers, clients, past coaches, and leaders in the fitness and inspiration fields who have all helped remind me to remain a student. You have all influenced me in ways you may not even know. Without you, I would have never become who I am today, and ForeverFitU would have never been born.

Thank you to all the ForeverFit folks who contributed to this book. You are an inspiration to all those striving to make fitness a lifestyle that lasts a lifetime. Thank you also to all of the ForeverFit individuals that I didn't get to interview. Continue to be the leaders of health for all those around you.

Thank you to you, the reader. Reading this book means you care enough about yourself to take positive steps toward a better tomorrow and toward the rest of your life. Forever begins now!

CHAPTER 1

The Power of Permanent Change

"Things do not change, we change."
Henry David Thoreau

"It may be hard for an egg to turn into a bird; it would be a jolly
sight harder for it to learn to fly while remaining an egg. We are
like eggs at present. And you cannot go on indefinitely being
just an ordinary, decent egg. We must be hatched or go bad."
C.S. Lewis

In a *Fast Company* article titled "Change or Die," Dr. Merzenich showed in a study how, after two hundred repetitions, a rat could learn to solve a puzzle and was then able to remember how to solve it for nearly the rest of its life. Essentially, by repetition, the rat had actually changed its brain. Becoming ForeverFit is as much about changing your brain as it is about changing what you do physically.

You are about to make a journey to change. Understand that there is no better time than now to do so. Have you been the egg described in C.S. Lewis's quote? Is it time for you to hatch? As you read this chapter, remember you are an egg that is beginning to hatch, and it is all right if you cannot fly just yet. Let hatching be good enough for now. You will fly eventually.

Understanding these stages of change will significantly help you to become ForeverFit. Change is really nothing more than learning something new. We all remember learning to read, write, ride a bike, drive a car, learn a new language, etc. Regardless of what you are learning, the process is the same. The goal here is to understand the process of change so you know that what you are going through is normal. We have all created unconscious habits in our lives. The power comes from understanding how these habits form. Once you understand that, you have the power to become ForeverFit. Below, I will illustrate the stages of becoming ForeverFit by comparing them with learning to drive a car. It is your job to figure out where you are on this continuum and to decide what you need to do to get to the next stage, which I will map out for you. The four basic stages are as follows:

- **Unaware**
- **Aware**
- **Prepare (and Act)**
- **You Are There!**

Stage 1: Unaware. In this stage, you do not even know there is a problem—you are in denial. In our learning-to-drive-the-car example, this is when you are in a car seat and probably don't understand what a car is. In this stage, you will never make an effort to learn. You are unaware. You have to become aware that the possibility of driving even exists before you will begin to think about ways you will do it. In this example, this stage is relatively short lived.

Those in this stage of the ForeverFit journey usually aren't exercising because they are somewhat ignorant. They often have no idea of the health issues brought on by not exercising. They also have no idea of the energy, vitality, and confidence they could get from exercising. They know what exercise is; they just don't know that many of the problems they are experiencing have anything to do with it (other than maybe being overweight). Exercise is, therefore, something that is a burden, and thus, something they avoid even thinking about. Many in this stage are also in denial; they may even lie to others about their exercise habits (or lack thereof). To get to Stage 2, these people need education, either from a book such as this, articles on fitness and health, or from an expert they trust that can show them there is hope. They also need to hear stories of those who are in the situation they are in that have overcome it through exercise. Those who are in denial simply need to be ready. Unfortunately, this often happens after things like heart attacks and the diagnosis of degenerative diseases.

If you know anyone in this stage, be a good friend. Get them some solid information on the benefits of exercise. Have them get some blood work done. Let them know you care about their health and want them to live a full, vibrant life.

Stage 2: Aware. In this stage, you become aware the problem exists, but still have no idea how you are going to fix it. You, therefore, begin to take steps to figure out a solution. You read up on it, ask family and friends about it, and when it pops up in the news, you are all ears. This is like the child who realizes big people drive cars and begins to wonder why children can't drive. They may even ask, "Can I drive?" or, heaven forbid, try driving on their own, obviously with no success. Many accept the fact that they can't drive now and wait until a later date. From here, they may inquire about wanting a tricycle, bicycle, four-wheeler, or one of those $300 Hummers for kids—*they want to drive!*

A good percentage of people on the ForeverFit path are in this stage. Many are sick and tired of where they are and have decided to educate themselves. Like the child wanting to drive, they want to get on an exercise program, one they can stick to, but have no idea what to do or how they are going to do it. Some actually go right to the next stage of trying something, which often leads to frustration and failure. To get to Stage 3, you need one or two things: proper guidance and/or motivation. Here are a few suggestions for both.

Find a good personal trainer

Finding a trainer or accountability partner you can trust to keep you on the proper path can help you immensely in getting to the next stage of change. A good trainer needs to be able to put you on a systematic, progressive program you can stick to long term and help you up when you fall the first few (or few dozen) times. He or she also needs to let you make your own mistakes and learn from them, kind of like raising children. If we do everything for our children, they never grow as they should. On my website (www.foreverfitu.com) is a list of key questions you can ask when hiring a personal trainer that can really help you in making the proper choice. As of this writing, the personal training industry is too unregulated, and I want you to get the most out of your personal training experience by choosing a trainer that has the proper background and experience to deliver what you need.

If there was anything in life you wanted to learn, you looked for a good instructor to teach you, correct? We hire accountants to do our taxes, carpenters to remodel our homes, and plumbers to fix leaky faucets. So why not hire someone, at least on a periodic basis, to look after and design your long-term fitness program? Notice I said on a *periodic* basis. If you are doing your part, you do not have to see your trainer two to three times per week. But I would suggest seeing him or her more often at the beginning to help you establish your exercise habit and start a roadmap of success. If you aren't planning on working with your trainer long term, please do yourself a favor and wean yourself off of him or her. In my experience, those who go from working with a trainer two to three times per week to zero all have quit within weeks to months.

If, after you decide you no longer need a trainer but aren't 100 percent confident you can do it on your own yet, see your trainer periodically to keep the accountability factor in play. If you enjoy working with your trainer, can afford it, and your trainer is giving you what you need, keep working with him or her. For example, many of my ForeverFit clients I've been working with for seven to ten years still have appointments with me once per week, or as little as once per month. Just make sure that part of your training sessions includes talking about your exercise habits outside of working together. Accountability is very important, especially at first, so having a regular appointment will help keep you accountable between training sessions.

If you want to get past Stage 2, seek help. Good trainers are out there. Seek and ye shall find. The Internet is a useful tool for finding a trainer. Some trainers even do online training for a cheaper fee, as well as phone consultations if you are in an area without a fitness facility. Not seeking out a fitness professional would be like reading a book on how to drive and trying to drive without having an instructor there beside you at first, guiding you. You may eventually figure out how to drive, but it will take a lot longer and you may crash a lot more before you figure it out.

Join a group

So what do you do if you can't afford a trainer? Try group training! You can cut your training cost 50 to 90 percent by splitting the fees with the others in your group. The group dynamic also provides extra motivation. It's more fun, and you have accountability partners! I have been working with groups since the year 2000, and my group members tell me how it motivates them to come to their group sessions.

If you already are motivated and simply need some structure, do your research and find good books or DVDs on fitness. Research online, ask a fitness professional, or ask someone who is ForeverFit where they learned what to do. The bottom line in Stage 2 is that if you need education, you need to find some. If you need motivation, read on.

Stage 3: Prepare (and act). In this stage, the person is preparing for action and actually begins to take action. This is the teenager who begins driver's education and behind-the-wheel training, yet isn't ready to be on his or her own yet. They are doing all of the preparation for the real thing by educating themselves and working with someone who knows how to drive and knows the rules to follow. You can probably remember this stage when you had to think about every little thing—placing hands at ten and two o'clock, accelerating too fast, braking too late, and riding the clutch, killing the engine. Everything is an effort to keep the vehicle in some type of control. It's no wonder the behind-the-wheel instructor has a brake on his or her side! You are getting better at the skill, but just aren't ready to be on your own yet.

Those in stage 3 compose another relatively high percentage of ForeverFit seekers, but for many this is often short lived. These folks have hired the trainer and/or have been reading up on all of the fitness articles (done the preparation), yet are still struggling with making it to the gym and/or are struggling outside of their sessions with their trainer. Although they are struggling, some keep going, while others fall to the wayside. As I mentioned before, there is nothing wrong with being in this stage, if you can afford it and are happy there (some of my clients are there, are happy, and are getting great results). However, if you want to get to stage 4 or if you want to change how you are doing outside of working with your trainer, you need merely two things—repetition and practice.

How did you make activities such as talking, reading, writing, spelling, riding a bike, and brushing your teeth an unconscious act? By doing it over and over and over and over and over again. For many years I brushed my teeth consistently but failed to be consistent at flossing. Why? Laziness? Hardly. Flossing takes practically the same physical effort as brushing. It is simply because I had brushed consistently longer than flossing, so brushing had become normal. Now that I have been educated more about the benefits of flossing, and understand these stages of change, I floss much more consistently. I may slip back again, and if I do, I know I will get back into the habit by simply repeating this habit more often. Since this works for everything else that has become normal for you, why not use the same strategy for making exercise feel like a normal part of your life? It never will until it has been done consistently long enough.

How Often to Exercise

You may ask, "How many days a week should I exercise?" Although this is a loaded question due to goals, etc., I suggest doing something active every day, especially at the beginning. Reading this chapter, you can understand why. The more days you consciously take time to do something active, the closer you are getting to making it a habit. Even a fifteen-minute walk during your lunch break (that you normally wouldn't do) is fine. It is the conscious mental effort of taking time out of your busy day to exercise that is as important as physically doing the exercise. By doing this, you are saying to yourself, "Exercise is important to me."

In this stage, those who slip back have failed at one of two things: preparation or action. Psychologist and author Nathanial Branden stated, "A goal without an action plan is a daydream." Having a goal, yet no action plan to complete the goal, is exactly what many do. They know where they want to be, yet may have jumped right into this phase with no guidance or preparation. Then they get too sore, get injured, feel stupid because they don't know what they are doing, fall victim to intimidation, don't get results in two weeks like the infomercials have been telling them all their lives, etc. Because of their lack of education, guidance, and preparation, they soon fall back into their old ways, often due to simple frustration.

The other person in stage 3 who slips back simply takes no action. He or she has all the intention and has mapped everything out, yet he or she does not take that first big step forward. If you lack preparation, prepare. If you lack action, do something to get started. Wherever you may lie in this spectrum, read on. There are chapters for you later in *ForeverFitU*.

I will give you tools to help you stick with exercise long enough so you won't have to consciously think about doing it any longer. But what if you did? Would that be such a horrible thing, having to think about things that keep you healthy, looking good, feeling good, and having more energy? Getting to the final stage is just a matter of time. How long it takes depends on consistency, repetition, desire, commitment, and a strong understanding of why you're doing it—all of which can be worked on and will be addressed in *ForeverFitU*.

Stage 4: You're there! In this final stage, you do the behavior all the time and never really have to think about it or plan it. It is something you just do. It has become part of you. A few weeks or months after getting your driver's license, you can drive with one hand on the wheel while talking on your cell phone or having your arm around your significant other. This is obviously not a safe way to drive, but you get the idea. How does this happen? Repetition. There is no conscious thought to what you are doing because you have been doing it so much. The level of unawareness you reach in any skill has to do with how many times you have repeated it, nothing else. Some actions become subconscious quickly, while others take some time.

I remember how hard parallel parking was when I first started driving (I actually failed that part of my driver's test). Because I was so bad at it, I avoided it, and guess what? I stayed bad at it! It wasn't until I decided to start doing it anyway that it became much easier, and now I don't think about it at all; I just do it. This may not be the case for your parallel parking skills, but you get the point. Repetition is the key to reaching this final stage. The number of repetitions required is different for everyone, but repetition is essential.

One thing that can help you reach and eventually stay in this final stage is to read the following paragraph that describes those in this stage, where the ForeverFit people reside. Doing so repeatedly will etch a picture in your mind of who you intend to be, and your actions will soon follow.

This group is probably reading this book to confirm why they do what they do on a daily basis. To these people, exercise has become such a part of their lives that their lives revolve around it. They know that exercise not only keeps them looking better, but, more importantly, it keeps them feeling better. When they are up, they work out in order to keep feeling up. When they are down or depressed, they work out harder, knowing they will feel much better afterward. When times are tough, the last thing they will let go of is their exercise because it is the one thing that will help keep them strong physically, mentally, and spiritually. To these folks, there is no substitute to exercise. It has become a permanent part of daily life. Exercise and health is a top priority to them and their actions show it. They may get thrown off track by major life events, illness, or injury, but it is very short lived and they have an understanding that they are coming back. It never leaves their consciousness. It is just something they do, no questions asked, no thinking or planning when to exercise (for the most part). Although it is still a choice, it has become an subconscious one. These people are the envy, and now the inspiration, of many.

Each of these stages could take years to reach, or it could happen in moments. When it happens in a moment, say a huge thank you. If it seems to be taking years, don't worry. All that matters is that you are taking steps to get to the next stage.

Dr. James Prochaska, a psychologist, found that roughly half of those who started a New Year's resolution had quit after one month. In this fifteen-year study of over sixty thousand people he found that one of the biggest reasons people didn't succeed in keeping their resolutions is that they didn't understand the stages of change, and when they fell off the horse the first time, they quit rather than seeing it as simply part of the process. Falling off the horse is no big deal. Not getting back on again, however, is. Or, as the great coach Vince Lombardi said, "It's not whether you get knocked down, it's whether you get up." Understanding change this way can dramatically help you become ForeverFit. It will make the bumps in the road less bumpy. Just understand that change is a process, not a destination.

Dr. Prochaska prefers to call this shifting between stages recycling verses relapsing, stating that this recycling is just part of the process for most people. He found that only about 5 percent of people actually went from one end of change to the other without recycling. So don't be concerned if you recycle. Just become aware of it and take the necessary steps to get back on track. At the same time, don't think that you can't be one of the 5 percent. Since it does happen, why shouldn't it happen to you?

A good thing about reaching the final stage is that if you can get there, you are much less likely to ever slip all the way back into the first stage of not even thinking of exercising. This is another great reason to get to this final "You are there!" stage. I can tell you from witnessing many clients over the years that this recycling of stages is true for most.

("FF" will be the abbreviation I use for ForeverFit. The following sentence has "FF 28." This depicts how many years that this person has been exercising consistently—28 years for Cheryl.)

Cheryl (FF 28) had a five-year span where she got off track, from age forty to about forty-five, because she traveled for work and was raising five teenagers. During this time, however, she never quit thinking about exercise. When it was time to get exercising again, she decided to seek out a personal trainer. She has been ForeverFit again for more than ten years and intends to stay that way. She keeps working with me, knowing that it is needed for her strength training and her "psychotherapy." Don't worry if the progress you are making toward becoming ForeverFit is a wavy line. Just stay on the line, and you will be fine.

Fear of Change

One big reason people fail at change is fear—fear of change and fear of success. Dr. Denis Waitley, a world-renowned motivational speaker who has worked with Super Bowl and Olympic athletes, Apollo astronauts, and top Fortune 500 executives, states that we often fear change due to being too comfortable in some of our current habits. He says that the best way to break out of your comfort zone is to take risks. These risks aren't really risky, though. They may include taking a different way to work, spending time in cultures different from the ones we are accustomed to, or changing the way and places we vacation. He says to "embrace challenges with knowledge and adventure." He also states that we need to deem ourselves worthy of great things, and, "when [we] talk to [ourselves], do so with great respect."

Begin to embrace this journey of becoming ForeverFit with a sense of challenge and adventure rather than one of "What if I don't succeed?" Doing so will put you in a state of joy, which will in turn give you more energy to not only exercise, but to enjoy it more.

Is everything about you the same as it was ten, twenty, or thirty years ago? It sure isn't for me. We are all changing; only some of the changes we have to start ourselves. Change is inevitable, so why not take control of as much change as you can?

A great question to ask

One of the things to ask yourself is: "Am I willing to do what it takes to get to stage 4, or am I okay with having someone or something motivate me on a daily, weekly, or monthly basis?" There is not a wrong answer here. Just make sure you are truly happy where you are. If you decide it is time for the move, one thing you need to do is discover what sets these ForeverFit (FF) individuals apart from the rest. What reasons other than simple repetition has made them ForeverFit while most struggle? The following chapters will reveal these secrets and will give you things you can do on a daily basis to make your thoughts and actions change for the better.

We will start with the other five "P"owers that these people have that have made and kept them ForeverFit. Any of these powers they do not think they use are the ones that are so innate that they do not even know they have them, which is why I call them secrets. Remember that the only reason you do not have them is because you either haven't become conscious of them yet, or you haven't repeated them enough. Do so and you will have them as well.

Applying the Power of Permanent Change to Becoming ForeverFit

1. Become aware of what needs to change.
2. Plan and take action. Find someone or something to help you.
3. Repeat the actions until they become unconscious acts.
4. Look at becoming ForeverFit as a fun challenge and an adventure.

CHAPTER 2

The Power of Practice

"Practice is the best master."
Latin proverb

"Energy and persistence conquer all things."
Benjamin Franklin

Why is practice the "best master"? Simply because whatever you practice, whether it be physically or mentally, you will soon become. If you were to ask most professional athletes or actors at the top of their game about how they prepare for their sport or performance, they would tell you about how hard they work at not only physically practicing their skills, but also mentally preparing for their upcoming events. When Jim Carrey was a child he would see how many ways he could contort his face in the mirror. I'd say it paid off.

In this chapter, you'll learn how to make not only physical practice, but also mental practice, work for you. And I'll share my secret to getting started and making progress. It's essential gear for your journey to becoming ForeverFit.

Practice for Permanence and Normalcy

We all have heard the phrase "practice makes perfect," which I consider to be an illusion. Do professional athletes practice to become perfect? Hardly. Life, like sport, is not perfect. So why should we try to be perfect when it comes to our exercise habits?

I prefer the phrase "practice makes permanent" because permanence is what happens when you practice anything long enough. It becomes more and more a part of you. The more permanent your new habits become, the more confident you become. The more confident you become, the more positive habits you will add to your life, including becoming ForeverFit.

You are what you practice on a daily basis. Both your good and bad habits become permanent. If you practice watching TV and eating chips, you'll get very good at it—and your body and mind will reflect that habit. If you practice going for an early morning walk, you'll get good at that. And you'll reap the mental and physical benefits.

This concept of practice is often overlooked, especially in exercise books. Many books and videos show you all of the exercise routines, which is great and obviously essential, yet they never say how long to practice it until it feels like a more natural part of your life.

Infomercials do exactly the opposite. They promise you a firm, toned body in as little as *x* number of weeks. Or they promise that you will lose up to *x* number of pounds or take as much as *x* number of inches off your waist. Do you realize that even if you lose no weight and take no inches off your waist, you have still lost *up to* x pounds and have lost *as much as* x inches off your waist?

Many people fall for these alluring promises of quick fixes. Then they become frustrated after the first few weeks and quit. If you've tried this, you know exactly what I'm talking about. The excitement of the new routine fades as the 25-plus pounds you gained in the last ten years aren't melting away. You feel cheated. Or you decide this stuff just doesn't work for you. This is one huge reason that a majority of people quit their exercise routines within the first two months. They haven't been told that it often takes months to years for exercise to feel like a normal part of life. The ForeverFit people I interviewed confirmed this. They also haven't been taught the importance of nutrition combined with exercise when it comes to becoming your ideal weight. Those of you who desire to become your ideal weight, please do yourself a favor and get help with your nutrition. It is a huge part of changing your weight for the better.

That's not a message that many of the quick-fix people want to deliver. But I'm delivering this message to you because you need to know it. Here's the honest truth: Exercise will only feel normal for you after you have done it consistently long enough.

Steve (FF 28) knows all about this. For the first eight years of Steve's fitness career, he was inconsistent for many reasons. He claims that it wasn't until he began running *every* night after college that exercise began to feel like a normal part of his life. During the eight years that Steve didn't work out every night, he was still exercising; it just didn't feel normal—essential—to him yet.

Steve's story drives home two huge points. First, it doesn't matter how long it takes for regular physical activity to feel normal. Just keep exercising! His story also underscores the value of repetition. Exercise in some way every day, even if it's only a five-minute walk or a few stretches at bedtime, and it will begin to feel normal to you much more quickly than if you do a big workout once or twice a week but don't look for opportunities to be active outside of your official workout times.

The payoff is huge. At forty-one, Steve now sees exercise as an incredible privilege to have in his life. Steve's philosophy when it comes to exercise is best summed up by a quote he gave me: "Life's journey is not to be laid to rest in a well-preserved body, but rather to come screaming in sideways, yelling, 'Holy crap, what a ride!'" He has obviously got the attitude thing down.

Knowing that exercising will probably not feel normal to you right away is very powerful for many reasons. First, you will start to think more long term. Second, when you hit bumps in the road (which you certainly will), or you have a bad week you will realize this is just part of the practice, like learning to ride a bike and falling off at first. Third, that annoying feeling of having to force yourself to exercise will be okay. Why? Because you will know that one day it won't feel like forcing any more if you just keep practicing.

Then one day it happens. You wake up in the morning and ask yourself, "When am I going to work out today?" *before* you think of all the other stuff you have to do. Get here and you have begun the shift to making physical activity a normal part of your life.

The coolest thing is that you do not have to wait for this day to come after weeks or months of practicing. You can make it happen now. In chapters 4 and 5 you will discover what you can do to shift your thinking in this direction. What is going to help you make this shift to thinking about exercise before other things occur? Practice, practice, practice.

For the golfer to learn a new swing technique, he or she needs to hit over two thousand balls while consciously thinking about this change before it will begin to feel normal and natural. Regardless of whether it is five hundred or five thousand swings, the point is that it needs to happen more than just at the lesson.

As you begin your journey of becoming ForeverFit, your new mantra is *practice*. Each and every day that you make positive steps toward your health and fitness is a practice day. Understand they are *all* practice days, not game days. No pressure. If you screw up, it's no big deal, because you are not in a game situation. In fact, the game never comes unless you decide to return to a sport you once loved, or to take up a new sport, or decide to do cycling rides, running races, triathlons, or other events. (I would recommend trying any or all if you are interested.) If you decide to try any kind of sport or event, your practice will become even more meaningful and fun.

My Secret: the Morning Meeting

Exercising itself is one component of practice. You must physically perform the act if you ever want to get better at it and have it feel like a normal activity for your body. The other equally important aspect of practice is the mental game you play with yourself on a daily basis: your constant self-talk. Physical activity has a definite start and stop time. However, your self-talk doesn't.

If you are asking yourself "What is this self-talk thing?" you have actually just discovered it by asking yourself that question. Self-talk is that constant voice inside you that is thinking, analyzing, criticizing, and worrying. You know the one. Unfortunately, unless you retrain it, your self-talk rarely pushes you in a positive direction. Instead, self-talk specializes in putdowns, doubts, and "you can't" messages.

Shifting your self-talk from destructive to productive patterns is very powerful, since this voice rarely (if ever) turns off. To begin to change your self-talk, you have to become aware of it first. You do this by catching yourself when you notice certain thoughts or actions arise in your mind.

How do you do that? Here's my simple and powerful secret. It changed my life, and I hope it will change yours. Introduce the Morning Meeting into your life.

Your Morning Meeting is a brief appointment you make with yourself first thing in the morning. It will only take a few minutes; so don't worry about those last few moments of sleep. Trust me: Morning Meetings will give you a lot more energy and help you become ForeverFit much more effectively than five to ten minutes of sleep could ever do. Why? Because this is when you shift your thinking into influencing your daily actions.

I can feel your skepticism as I write this. You're probably saying, "Right. It's hard enough to get up now. How can I make myself get up even earlier? And what exactly do I do with this time? How could this really make such a big difference?" Well, to find out if the Morning Meeting works for you, you'll just have to do it. I have developed a Morning Meeting Manual to help guide you through this process more easily. Here are my six instructions for success.

1. Set your alarm for an odd time.

If you usually get up at 6:00a.m., set your alarm for 5:47 or 5:53 or however much time you need. This odd time will help remind you of your Morning Meeting for the first few weeks. Don't get up with the *exact* amount of time it takes to do your meeting, however. Give yourself a little extra time so you can really contemplate what you are working on. It is important to *feel* what it is you are reading to yourself and thinking about, so make sure your Morning Meeting doesn't become some boring routine you do. One thing to do is have a variety of quotes and sayings that inspire the start of your day.

2. Smile and say thank you for another day of practice.

It doesn't have to be a big grin. Try a half smile and see what happens to your mind and your emotions. Your smile must be sincere for your Morning Meeting to be effective. If you are smiling, but inside you are saying "Why do I have to do this?" or "I can't believe it is time to get up," your mind will not be nearly as receptive to the thoughts you are going to feed it. Saying a big thank you is also important, because it starts your mind on a positive track. You're noticing and appreciating the pluses in your life (rather than dwelling on the problems or worries). That gets your daily self-talk off to a healthy start.

3. Read and write to reinforce your positive self-talk.

Spend the next few minutes reading a passage that inspires you and is pertinent to the goal you are working on in your fitness life. (If possible, read aloud. Abraham Lincoln found that he remembered twice as much when he read aloud, and I agree with him.) Reflect on what you learned from previous days. Have a small notepad handy to write down what you learned from each day (especially the bad ones). This will help you identify what could have worked better. Throughout the book I will give you suggestions of things to work on during your Morning Meetings. The Morning Meeting Manual (MMM) will chart out exactly what to do and how to do it to make this meeting work for you.

Below are a few examples of different individuals and what they might include at their Morning Meetings. Remember, this meeting will constantly change as you accomplish certain things and when other issues arise. Remember not to focus on the problem. Instead focus on the solution to it. Focusing on the problem will only create more problems. Focusing on the solution is the only way to create a solution. Sounds simple, yet it is a *huge* concept to grasp and utilize when constructing your Morning Meeting.

Example 1: Mary, mother of three young children, is looking to get back in shape after having babies.

Issue: It is difficult to find time to exercise while taking care of three young children; she's tired all the time.

Morning Meeting: "I will make time today for exercise because of its importance in my life. Even if it means I have to get up twenty to thirty minutes earlier, I will do it! I want to be an example to my children by showing them that exercise is an important part of life so if I have to do it during my day, I will tell them that this is Mommy's time to exercise. I will make it a normal part of our day. I know that exercise will only add to my energy, and as soon as I get going I will be fine."

Example 2: Joe is a middle-aged man who has been on and off the exercise wagon for years and is ready to make a permanent change.

Issue: He isn't sure how he is going to break this chain of inconsistency.

Morning Meeting: "What things can I do today to make sure I get my workout in?" Read things like "Today is the most important day to exercise" and "I am a consistent exerciser." Then he can visualize and really feel as if he is ForeverFit.

Example 3: Suzie has put on forty pounds in the last ten years.

Issue: She wants to get back to her original weight in the next six months.

Morning Meeting: Tape a picture of herself at her original weight on or inside her Morning Meeting Manual (MMM), along with the weight she desires to be and the date at which she wishes to be that weight. She can ask a question like "What will I feel like when I am back to that weight?" From here she might simply meditate on this feeling as she gets ready for her day.

4. Keep it simple.

You probably have enough going on in your life that you don't need to bog yourself down with ten mental fitness goals to work on every day. Just pick one or two things, such as a goal, a thought, a new attitude, or practical strategy, to practice at a time.

For example, if your current stumbling block is your old belief "I'll never stick with exercise, so why bother trying?" then, in your Morning Meeting, you should reread one or two of the FF profiles that inspire you. Write down a new phrase you're going to substitute every time your mind sends you your old belief. Maybe it's "I don't know if I can do it forever, but I am going to do it today." Maybe it's "If Susan can do it, I can do it!" (See Chapter 3) Or "I can and I will make this change, one day at a time." You get the idea.

5. Carry your meeting into your day.

You can think about what you read and wrote and thought as you are showering and getting ready for your day. If you become a morning exerciser, go over your Morning Meeting as you exercise! Letting your positive self-talk become part of your day can dramatically increase the Morning Meeting's effect.

6. Repeat.

This daily appointment is crucial for your long-term success, and repetition is the key. If you have been practicing sedentary living or sporadic exercise habits for many years, the only way to break this pattern permanently is to develop a new mind-set toward the role of physical activity in your life. The Morning Meeting helps you accomplish the absolutely necessary mind-set change you need to become ForeverFit.

You'll be amazed at the power of the Morning Meeting. I have used this Morning Meeting myself to help with many things that I felt needed a change. By starting my day looking at previous days and seeing what I would like to become as a father, I have seen my parenting improve dramatically. I have become much more patient with my boys, and when I do things or say things I wish I wouldn't have, the next morning I think how I will act the next time it comes up, and over time my actions changed. Some changed slower than others, but they did improve.

My Morning Meeting has also helped me minimize the consumption of caffeine, which had been a problem for me for years. I actually accomplished this using the stages of change I mentioned earlier, as well as other concepts you will learn in this book. This, in turn, made me less irritable and actually *increased* my energy. These are only a couple things that the Morning Meeting has helped me with, and I am constantly working on others. If becoming ForeverFit is important enough to you, begin this meeting and watch what it will do for your exercise habits.

Once the Morning Meeting becomes an automatic start to your day, you have created a powerful ally. Just like all habits, it will become more automatic the more often you do it, so do it every day if possible. Eventually you will crave it because of its positive effect on your day and life. You'll be able to watch the snowball effect of personal growth for you. Don't be surprised if the Morning Meeting starts to make your whole life go better as you create positive mental habits. The MMM will guide you and direct you along your path to becoming ForeverFit.

Use Daily Practice Reminders

Give yourself constant reminders about practicing throughout your day, especially for the first few weeks. Stick notes around the house, in your car, and at work with the word *practice* on them, or maybe just a big **P**. This will remind you throughout your day to **p**ractice what you really want in your fitness life. Those **P**s can also help remind you of the other five "**P**" powers mentioned later in this book: **p**ermanent change, **p**erspective, **p**riority, **p**roper questions, and **p**ictures. One way to do it: Go to a craft store and get a bunch of sticky letter **P**s. Put them on your bathroom mirror, your briefcase, the dashboard of your car, gym bag, or whatever you use on a daily basis. Stick one or two **P**s on your fridge, too, especially if you are also working on nutrition.

Here's the best news: When you combine the Morning Meeting with **p**ositive mental self-talk throughout the day, your **p**hysical change will come even faster. We all look for quick fixes. Becoming ForeverFit isn't a quick-fix solution, but using these two tools—the Morning Meeting and mental **p**ractice—will accelerate your **p**rogress, I **p**romise.

This may sound odd, but make sure you cut yourself a little slack from time to time. If you do not practice at all in a day once in awhile, that's okay. If you miss a day of practice, you won't backslide. Missing a couple of weeks or a month or a year is a whole different story.

Make it fun

Here's another tip that has worked for several ForeverFit folks: Make up games to help reinforce your practice. After all, practice is supposed to be fun, not a chore. One example of a game could be to pay yourself for your Morning Meeting or maybe for each time you go to the gym.

Even if it is one dollar at a time, attaching a monetary value can help make practice more fun and you get an instant reward, even if it is a small one. Paying yourself and watching your paycheck grow can be a good symbol of how many small steps can help you achieve a big goal over time.

Is money too tight to pay yourself? Use stickers on a calendar as a visual measure of your efforts. Or make yourself a chart on which you can mark your progress. Post a map and make imaginary trips, translating workout times or miles (or morning meetings) into miles on a journey. For example, one hour of exercise could equal 60 miles. You can head to the Grand Canyon, or Alaska, or Palm Beach. You get the idea.

Other free ideas would be to meet a friend for a walk, a bike ride, or check out whatever free event in your area appeals to you. The point is to do something you enjoy, something you wouldn't normally do (that doesn't revolve around food).

The bottom line: Becoming ForeverFit starts in your head

Mental practice is at least as important as the physical act of exercising. As Ralph Waldo Emerson wisely stated, "The ancestor of every action is a thought." In other words, wherever your thoughts are going, you can bet your bottom dollar your actions are about to go in that direction too. So make your thoughts work for you, not against you.

To make sure you get your Morning Meeting in every day, first of all you must believe in its value. The only way to truly believe in something is to have direct experience of it. If you understand the power of repetition by now, this should help you to begin to believe in the value of this meeting, but it will never get you all the way to believing in its value until you experience it for yourself. So now make it work for you. Wake up at an odd time. Put your Morning Meeting Manual or notebook somewhere where you have to move it to do some other early morning tasks: on top of your toothpaste, or right in front of your pills. Maybe even set it on top of your alarm clock. If you are a person who likes to check off tasks you've completed, put the Morning Meeting in your daily scheduler or blackberry. Start your day in the right direction. See where it takes you.

Be ready to go

The Morning Meeting and mental preparation won't help in the long run unless you actually get your workout in. That means you are ready to make it happen when you have the time. I strongly recommend you have your gym bag somewhere you will see it, preferably on top of some other stuff you have to do, to remind yourself to exercise first. Pack your bag the night before and perhaps set it in the doorway to your bathroom or in front of your bedroom door; somewhere where it will get in your way.

The same principle applies if you are planning to run or bike from home. Get your clothes and gear out the night before and put them where you can't possibly miss them. Then you won't fall prey to the well-known 6:00 a.m. copout: "I would do it, but I don't know where my (insert missing item here) is."

Many FF people schedule their workouts in their schedule book or blackberry. Cheryl (FF 28) says she has to schedule her workout or she won't do it. That's why she believes a personal trainer has been so good for her. It is an appointment she knows she needs to keep.

Suzanne (FF 23) uses a calendar in which she writes in her training times each week. She says looking at the calendar helps remind her of her planned commitment to exercise. It also reminds her what she intends to do in each session (walk, swim, strength training, etc.).

You could set an alarm to go off thirty minutes after work is over. That can be your reminder to head out for your run, walk, bike ride, or whatever you have planned for that day. You could also post a sticky note in your cube at work every Monday morning. That becomes your draft activity list for the week. You can then check off or substitute activities as you complete them throughout the week.

Applying practice to your ForeverFit goal

1. Schedule your Morning Meeting every morning at an odd time, give yourself ample time to do it, and put your notebook or Morning Meeting Manual in a place where you will see it.
2. Post reminders at home and work that prompt you to practice, both physically and mentally.
3. Make practice fun and rewarding. Do it often.

CHAPTER 3

The Power of Perspective

**"If you change the way you look at things, the
things you look at change."**
Albert Einstein

Everything has a perspective. This observation from Einstein
dealt with observing microscopic organisms. As you turn up the
magnification, the entire world you are looking at changes. Just as
microorganisms begin to look totally different as you look at them
with different magnifications, so do the circumstances of your life, if
you are willing to see them from another perspective. The following
story is not only inspiring, but offers a great example of how one's
perspective on a very bad situation has yielded incredibly positive,
long-term results. Susan Peters' story has positively impacted many
other lives, and now yours.

Susan's Story

Susan Peters' vehicle got crushed between a street sander and
another automobile in a winter storm in December 1993, leaving her
in a coma for three months. The doctors told her family that if she
regained consciousness, she would be a vegetable, like the woman
many of us remember, Terry Schiavo. They said she would never
be able to walk, talk, or feed herself again, not to mention perform
other basic daily activities. Many surgeries later, due to a poor job of
splinting in her arms and hands, she was told that not only would

she never walk again, but she would have extremely limited use of her arms and hands.

Susan didn't believe a single word they said. She decided it was her job to not only walk again, but also to get her driver's license, ride her horses again, lift weights, and do all of the things she used to. For the next decade plus, she worked with physical therapists and personal trainers. Combining this with an amazing attitude, Susan got rid of her wheelchair and walked her first 5k (3.1 miles) in October of 2005 in 3 hours and 14 minutes. In October 2006, she completed the same 5k in 1 hour and 59 minutes!

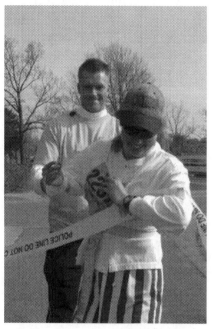

Susan would come to the gym, sometimes with black eyes, joking that she got in another fight at the bar, but we all knew what happened. She has no ability to catch herself when she falls and sometimes would go head first into the

Susan at the end of her first 5k with her trainer, Erik Peacock.

coffee table or edge of the couch. But, as Susan always did, she would joke about it. She realized at one point that the only way she was going to accelerate her walking skills was to get rid of her wheelchair at home, and she paid the price a few times. I had the pleasure of working with Susan every few months when her regular trainer was out of town, and I got to witness her drastic improvements through the years. I have seen her go from walking one-eighth of a mile in 45 minutes to doing a whole mile in less than that amount of time within a couple of years, and she is only getting faster. We used to have to hold on to what Susan referred to as her "fashion belt" (which is a strap around her waist that I would hang onto in case she lost her balance) when she walked, and she now gets up and walks from one room to the other on her own. The most amazing thing about Susan's journey is that she does everything with a smile on her face, laughing, joking, and never complaining. She even talks about her accident as "losing a game of chicken."

Susan's perspective on herself is not of someone who is handicapped, but is of someone who is getting better day by day, week by week, and month by month. She doesn't compare herself to others but, instead, compares how she was a month or year ago. She knows that it is her job to get better and is doing everything it takes to get there. This story is here to inspire you to take any excuses you feel you may have and find a way to shift perspective on them.

Below is something I wrote for Susan after her second 5k. It is something to offer you a little perspective in your own life and inspire you to make the most of what you have. It is something I feel that, if read every day, could give you the boost you need to keep going.

Susan,

Some of us listen to music, read books, pray, meditate, or look at the stars for inspiration. Others only need to watch you. You are an inspiration, Susan, not only because of your achievement today, but because of how you live your life. We all feel a connection with you, because deep down we all wish we could be more like you—always smiling, never complaining (even though you could complain about plenty), staring adversity and pain in the face and taking it head on. How do you do it? We all should have a picture of you to remind us not only of how much we have to be grateful for, but also how important attitude is in shaping our lives. You remind us of the power of the human spirit, and that when we think we can't change, that this is the way things always have been so that's the way they always will be, there is hope if we remember how you live—smiling through everything and keeping our perspectives and attitudes in check. You are proof that there is no limit to what we can accomplish, regardless of what the experts say. Thank you for your presence in our lives.

These words have been superimposed over a picture of Susan and a group of us that were with her at the finish of her second 5k. It is placed on a wall in the private studio that I work at for all to see and keep us reminded of what a great presence she has been in our lives.

These are only a few of the miraculous things Susan has done. She attempted to help her hands and arms by having weekly appointments with a physical therapist (that she referred to as a physical "terrorist") that would take an instrument basically like a butter knife and push it across her scar tissue to try to break it up and give her better range of motion. For her, the pain was nothing compared to what it was doing for her, especially since she had already been through more than a dozen surgeries. She is also only one of two people in her situation to have the baclofen pump removed. Baclofen is a drug that helped control spasticity in her muscles. She was the first, however, to have completely taken herself off the drug, due to the consistent personal training and physical therapy. She told me that the personal training helped her so much because it kept her brain active, making her think as exercises progressed and routines switched up.

I refer back to Susan's story often, because it fits into so much about what is written in ForeverFitU. It is obvious how her story fits into Perspective. It gives weight loss goals a whole new outlook, huh? This isn't to say that getting to a better weight isn't a worthwhile goal. Heck, even Susan has worked on dropping some weight, which she did. Changing perspective could just mean that if your goals aren't coming as fast as you would like, you can still be thankful for having a body that works, and that you can exercise. If you have been given the ability of movement, why not use it? Her story can also show you how taking the right perspective on tough times can help you grow.

Perspectives on setbacks and failing

Thinh Nhat Hanh, a nominee for the Nobel Peace Prize and author of over 25 books, had a great quote regarding perspective: "When I have a toothache, I discover that not having a toothache is a wonderful thing. That is peace." What a great perspective on pain and setbacks. Most of us, when encountering a setback, take the perspective of how awful it is. Looking at it from Hanh's perspective, we can see a positive in even the toughest of times. What if, while experiencing a setback, you saw it as an opportunity to be appreciative of the good times? I once saw on a T-shirt "Pain is just weakness leaving the body." Isn't this a much better way to view pain?

In the Bible it says to "give thanks in all circumstances" (1 Thessalonians 5:18, ESV). Why would you give thanks when bad things happen? Because when you do, your brain naturally shifts to the question "What can I learn from this?" This is a very powerful question to ask when something bad happens. So, you have two choices of how to use your past mistakes—to have something to feel guilty about or to learn from. Which do you think will help you become ForeverFit faster?

In strength training, a muscle only gets stronger through failure, yet most people believe failure is a bad thing. Failure is often that thing that propels you to another level if you see it as something to learn from rather than something to be upset about. Most people see their problems as something bad or something that shouldn't be happening. What if you saw every problem as a game of finding a solution? What if you saw every failure and setback as a chance to learn and grow? What if you saw every bad situation as a way to get perspective on those who have it worse?

None of us would ever learn and grow in life if it weren't for a fall or two. Don't regret that bad days happen. Instead, *learn from them.* Regretting that they happened helps nothing. Learning from setbacks accelerates growth. Since you can't go back and change your past actions, why not use them to assist you in the future? When you have a bad day or week of working out, let that teach you to be appreciative of those days and weeks that are good and that you are motivated. Always remember Susan's story. Read it at your Morning Meeting to remind yourself that things aren't all that bad, and if they are, what perspective can you take to help you learn from what you are going through that will propel you to a higher place?

Current beliefs

Pay attention to your current belief system since this is where a majority of your perspectives come from. All of the beliefs you carry with you are nothing more than thoughts you have been told over and over by others or have thought over and over to yourself, or from past experiences. Some of these beliefs have helped you in your life while others have not. The issue is that some of the beliefs that are limiting are so ingrained that you don't even know they are a belief, and you just accept them as reality when that may not be the case. Beliefs such as "creating healthy habits is hard," "I've always been this way so I will always be this way," or "I wasn't raised in a healthy environment so I have no choice as to my poor lifestyle habits" are beliefs that severely limit you in what you can accomplish. As a matter of fact, anything you label as an excuse is simply a limiting belief you have been telling yourself or others have been telling you for so long that it has become part of your belief system.

Having grown up in a Norwegian environment where the only color I ever saw on my plate was ketchup, I had a limiting belief that my sons wouldn't eat broccoli. But, my wife Meredith had grown up on all natural foods from the garden so her beliefs were different, and so were her actions. She cut the broccoli up into small pieces and made a game out of it, and the boys loved it! My limiting belief about broccoli carried over to the way I was feeding my children.

This concept is so important because you need to begin to pay attention to whom and what you are paying attention to. If you believe any of the limiting beliefs mentioned above or have excuses as to why you aren't ForeverFit, chances are someone who most likely wasn't ForeverFit has told them to you, or you are letting your past experiences control your current actions. Your beliefs are what you will act upon. So how do you go about changing these beliefs that limit you? The same way they were put there: by catching yourself when these beliefs creep in and replacing them with an empowering thought over and over until it becomes your new belief.

The key is in becoming aware of them, catching yourself, and in believing that the contents of this book will work for you. After all, if you believe they won't work for you, then that is the first belief you need to change, right? The biggest belief to shift off of is "this may work for others but will never work for me" or "I've never been able to stick to anything." Holding onto beliefs such as these will guarantee failure, since you will act upon these limiting beliefs. If you believe that because you have never been able to stick to anything and hold onto that belief, the first time you slip, you will say "See, there it goes again," and you will more than likely quit.

I would suggest putting the change of some of these limiting beliefs at the top of your Morning Meeting agenda. Reading these to yourself daily will change your belief system and, therefore, change your daily actions. A great example of how an ingrained belief can influence your actions is when you say how well something is going, have you ever knocked on wood? How automatically did this happen, and since when did wood have so much power? Did you really think your good fortune was going to go away if you didn't do it? Where did this belief come from?

Beliefs and the four-minute mile

As of May 5, 1954, no one had ever broken the four-minute mile. The previous record of four minutes, 1.4 seconds, had stood since 1945—nearly nine years passed without anyone being able to surpass this milestone. As a matter of fact, it was believed to be a physical human impossibility, like walking on the moon and climbing Mount Everest once were. The experts believed it would never be done without severe risk to the athlete. However, a man by the name of Roger Bannister believed something different. Rather than believing the experts, he asked, "What is a mere 1.4 seconds?" Through his belief in the possibility of a sub-four-minute mile (and obviously some great athleticism), he ran the mile in three minutes, 59.4 seconds on May 5, 1954. The amazing thing is that the conditions weren't even ideal. Within the next three years, sixteen runners broke the four-minute mile, and today thousands achieve it every year. What happened? Why did no one touch the previous record for nine years? Did humans suddenly evolve? Hardly. Their beliefs changed because they saw someone achieve it. As Roger Bannister proved, all you really have to do is change your belief first, and your actions will follow.

As your actions begin to change from these shifts in beliefs and you begin to see positive results from them, a snowball effect will begin and your beliefs will become reinforced. The FFs have reinforced their belief in the benefits of exercise so much that their belief has become a knowing. *Beliefs influence actions. Actions reinforce beliefs.* Remember this cycle. Choose which one to be on—limiting beliefs and limited action, or empowering beliefs and unlimited action. It's your choice.

Attitude is everything

Another thing that will dramatically affect your perspective is your attitude. Dr. Wayne Dyer said "There is no path to success; success is an inner attitude that we bring to our endeavors."

Charles Swindoll is a man I admire very much. His attitude quote is found all over the Internet and is something I intend to live by. He basically says there are many things in life that we cannot control, however attitude is not one of them. As a matter of fact, he says it is probably the most important choice we will make each and every day. Swindoll says, "I am convinced that life is 10 percent what happens to me and 90 percent how I react to it."

I would challenge you to make up an attitude quote of your own to use on a daily basis. See how many times every day that a shift in attitude changes your perception and therefore your actions on different situations. If you would like, take any or all of the attitude quote that I made for myself and use it as a starting point for you.

My Daily Attitude

Attitude is the most important choice I will make
every day.
Attitude will affect how I respond to whatever
comes at me today.
It will affect how I parent.
It will affect me as a husband.
It will affect me as a trainer, a coach, and a
businessperson.
It will affect how hard I exercise.

31

It will affect the foods I choose to eat.
It will affect me as a fellow human being.
Attitude comes from within, not from without.
My environment will not affect my attitude.
My attitude *will,* however, affect my environment.
I see every problem as a possibility.
I am grateful that I have the choice of which
attitude to choose today.
A shift in attitude is available to me at all times.
All I need to do is ask "What can I do to shift my
attitude right now?"
Today I choose the attitude of health, laughter,
gratitude, wisdom and love.

You will see the power of attitude in many of the stories you will read in *ForeverFitU*. Reading a quote like this one daily can help remind you that it isn't your circumstances that make you successful, but rather how you respond to your circumstances. So many of our reactions to life could be changed. For instance, if someone says something that offends us, we either judge them or respond with anger when we could respond with forgiveness and tolerance. We could understand that is where this person is right now in his or her life and hope that that person sees the light eventually. Too altruistic? Maybe, but it could be done. It is a choice.

You deserve this

The first attitude you must adopt is the attitude that you *deserve* to be ForeverFit. You owe it to yourself. You came into this world in a state of well-being, and it is God's intention you remain there. Regardless of your past, you deserve health and vitality. Exercise is one major component that can help you get more of both. Reading all of these secrets will help you a lot more if you feel you deserve to be ForeverFit. If you do not feel you deserve it, start now! Say it out loud to yourself: "I deserve to be ForeverFit!"

It is also your choice about how to respond to going through this book. What if you come in with the attitude that you will try anything if it might help? Have the attitude that this book ended up in your hands for a reason, and you intend to pay attention because there is wisdom here from those who are where you want to be. A great attitude is unstoppable. It is immune to the opinions of others, even the so-called experts. Have your attitude quote where you can see it often. It is the basis of every chapter in this book and a big key to becoming ForeverFit. Having a bad day? In a bad mood? Depressed? Feeling lazy? Kids driving you nuts? Read your attitude quote. You may find that it isn't that you had a bad day, but that you merely reacted to your day in a self-defeating way. Don't get mad that you did. Instead, take a look back and see how you could have reacted differently.

Banishing excuses

A great suggestion is to write down all excuses you have now or ever have had of why you don't exercise, and take a look at the ForeverFit person's perspective of them. For instance, do you really not have enough time, or do you choose to spend it in other ways? We all have 24 hours in a day. My typical clientele runs from as early as 6:00 a.m. to as late as 7:00 p.m. Monday through Friday with family obligations before and after work. I made a decision that the only way I was going to get my workouts in was to do them at or before 5:00 a.m. (if I didn't have any small breaks in my day). Just like anything, it was hard at first, but felt normal after doing it for six to nine months. Instead of being upset that I have to get up so early to exercise, I feel blessed to have this time for myself or to bond with my wife on the days we exercise together, and to be able to do this for myself and for us. The rest of the day is about doing things for everyone else, so this time is precious to me. I also don't feel cheated at the end of my day. I have made a decision to take this perspective. A perspective is just that: a decision.

Lack of time is just one of many excuses I hear as a trainer, most of which I have heard at one time or another in my twenty or more years as an avid exerciser. Although excuses make you feel safe because they don't force you to step out of your comfort zone, they also keep you right where you are. What are your excuses doing for you? What might happen if you shifted your perspective on them to those of the ForeverFit folks? Banishing excuses from your daily dialogue will help you stay motivated to become ForeverFit. I love what fitness guru Jack Lallane (FF 80+ when he passed away at age 96) said: "Too many people make excuses like 'I am too old,' or 'don't have the time,' or 'it costs money.' Then when they get sick they go to the doctor and want a shot in the backside to make them healthy." Below are other excuses and the ForeverFit person's perspectives on them. If any of these excuses apply to you, write down the new perspective and include it in your Morning Meeting so that you can be prepared to replace your old excuses with the new ForeverFit perspective the next time they creep in.

List of excuses and the FF perspective

1. I have too much stuff to do today/I don't have the time.

    FF perspective: I will be able to get done with all my stuff in a fraction of the time if I get my workout in because of the energy and focus it provides. If some of the stuff doesn't get done, that's okay. My workout comes first. By the way, why shouldn't my workout be part of my "too much stuff"? Steve (FF 28) says, "The correct phrase is *not* that you don't have the time, but that you choose to use your 24 hours to do everything but exercise. It is all about setting your priorities." Cathy (FF 5), mother of three children ages five and under, says, "You make the time day or night. I do not feel like I can get things done most days, so time could be my excuse, but I don't let it be if I want to feel good and have energy. You need to make the time for the things that mean the most to you."

2. I'm too stressed out.

    FF perspective: I am so stressed out that I need to work it off by exercising even harder. I know the endorphins that exercise provides will elevate my mood. Doris (FF 42) says she exercises "to keep myself physically strong to endure life's ups and downs."

3. I travel too much for my job.

FF perspective: I will find a way to get exercise in when I am on the road, even if it means I do a workout in my hotel room. Most hotels have fitness rooms with all my equipment needs at my disposal. If I need to, I will go on a walk, run, or climb the stairs of the hotel. Exercise is something that is too important to me to let slip because I'm not around my normal surroundings.

4. I'm too tired.

FF perspective: I may be tired, but I know that as soon as I get my blood flowing, I will be okay, say nothing about how I will feel afterward. All I have to do is get started and I will be fine. Mary (FF 27) says this excuse can be very real for some people. She says, "It's tough to convince someone who is exhausted that they will feel better if they exercise. Her suggestion: start with one small change. Get up ten minutes earlier to exercise or take a ten-minute walk at lunch, or go lift weights for ten minutes. Commit to doing that three times a week for three weeks and then see how you feel."

Kim (FF 24), a licensed psychologist, suggests giving yourself the "three-minute rule." This guideline goes like this: Commit to moving your body for three minutes, and then check in with your body to see if it still feels tired and doesn't want to move. If, however, after three minutes, your body decides it just needed a little warm-up and the movement feels good, you should continue with the exercise. She stresses that they *must* honor their body's desire to quit after three minutes if their body continues to say no to the exercise. If they don't, they will not create a healthy pattern that says, "I can trust myself."

5. My shoulder, back, knee, neck hurts.

FF perspective: the only way to make my joints feel better is to get them moving, so here I go. If exercise doesn't make them feel better, I will find a natural way to help them so that I can exercise better. Doris (FF 42) is seventy-seven years young and has back problems. She knows she must do certain exercises to keep it strong, and if she doesn't, her back tells her. Kim (FF 25) says to "find an exercise that works around the pain." I agree with her.

6. I don't have enough money to join a gym or hire a trainer.

FF perspective: I will cut out other things in my budget that aren't really doing me or my health any good in order to make joining a gym or hiring a trainer affordable. If I can't do that, I will buy a ball and exercise band and do in-home workouts for now. Either way, I will find a way to afford it. I only need to cut out less than two dollars a day to be able to join a gym. Marie (FF 45) states it very simply: "Too expensive? Plan your budget for it." If you still think it is too expensive, think about how expensive poor long-term health is. How expensive is it to not be able to do the things you once could? Expense isn't always in the form of money.

7. Exercise is just too hard.

FF perspective: It is much harder carrying around an extra twenty or more pounds and being out of breath and exhausted from doing mundane tasks your entire life than it is doing thirty to sixty minutes of exercise each day. Everything is hard when you first start it.

8. I feel too intimidated to go to a gym.

FF perspective: Intimidation is only from lack of knowledge or lack of experience. Everyone at the gym is so into their own workout that they don't have time to look at what I am doing. If I feel intimidated, however, I will educate myself on what to do or talk to a fitness professional I can trust. My fitness and health are much more important to me than what others think of me. Marie (FF 40) says, "I've *learned* not to care what other people say or how they look at me while [I'm] at the gym."

9. I feel too guilty taking time away from my family.

FF perspective: Exercise will only make me a better parent or spouse because of the de-stressing benefits and the energy it provides. My family knows how important it is to me and respects me for taking care of myself. The little time I take away from them to exercise is a bargain for what I get from it. I am also being a role model to my family by exercising. It is good for them to see the value of me taking care of myself. Also, there are plenty of ways we can exercise as a family that I could discover by merely searching the Internet for five minutes. Cathy (FF 5) says, "I have to be happy before I can make others happy."

10. I haven't lost any weight.

FF perspective: No matter what the result is on the scale, it will motivate me, otherwise I won't weigh myself. If I weigh in heavier than I wanted, it will motivate me to work even harder. If I weigh in lighter, it will motivate me to keep doing what I have been doing. If weighing myself is going to send me on an emotional roller coaster by what the number says, I am not using it to my advantage. I also know the value of proper nutrition and how it relates to body weight. I will seek out nutritional advice if I feel that I am doing all of the exercise I can and do not have the physical results I desire. Tim (FF 7) says the toughest part of staying in shape is "keeping going when you don't see any physical results." But you know what? He keeps going because he says that he has found things he likes to do, which makes it more enjoyable.

11. I don't know what to do.

FF perspective: If I feel I don't know what form of exercise to do, I will find someone or something to educate myself. I know how to walk, run, or bike.

Twenty degrees isn't that cold outside if it was ten below zero the day before. Put those twenty degrees in July and you have a different story. Wayne Dyer has very little hair on his head, but as he states, "If this was in a bowl of soup, this would be a lot of hair." Everything has a perspective. It is your choice of which one to choose. The rest of this book contains many more perspectives. See how changing your current one to the FF perspective will help you become ForeverFit.

Applying perspective to your ForeverFit goal

1. Everything has a different perspective if you are willing to look for it.

2. Change your perspective to how the FF person would see it if you want what they have, especially when excuses creep in.

3. Look at failure as something to learn from rather than something to be upset about.

4. Remember Susan's story and read it daily.

CHAPTER 4

The Power of Priority

"Action expresses priorities."
Mohandas Gandhi

As you shift perspective on things, your priorities will often naturally shift, as you will see in this chapter. This can shift both ways, however, so really watch your perspective.

My mid-twenties were the only time since I was thirteen years old that I took an extended break from consistent exercise. I got heavily involved in a business that shifted my priorities in life. This shift in priorities resulted from having the perspective that I could exercise again once I made all the money I needed. This may be typical of someone just getting out of college. My sole purpose and idea of success was how much money I could make, and this shift caused me to misalign my priorities. I exercised sporadically, lost twenty pounds of muscle and got a bigger belly, had no energy, and honestly had no real drive for life. I was a skinny guy with a belly. How is that possible?

I will never forget the day I decided to get back in the gym. I was driving a mail truck nine months later, jiggling my belly fat, and something just snapped. That day I joined the YMCA and never looked back. This was one example of slipping back a few stages of change and going from stage one to stage four in an instant. I told myself that exercise has to be a top priority in my life and always will have to be. It has been over a decade now, and I continue to be in the best shape of my life. This shift in priority was the biggest key for my success, as it is for many FF people.

Many people wonder how I can get up so early to exercise at that time of day. Proper prioritizing can help dramatically. Mary (FF 27) has four simple yet powerful words she says to herself in these early-morning hours to get herself out of bed and to the gym or out the door running: *"Don't think, just move."* I am in 100 percent agreement with this statement, simply because of the fact that the second you start thinking (unless you have conditioned yourself to give a smile and thanks for all of the things in your life), it usually won't come in a positive form. Instead, it usually comes in the form of all the reasons why you would rather stay in bed. These words are, as Mary said, time tested, so use them. I have, and they work.

Figure out a way to get it in and get it done

My older brother, Craig (FF 23), said, "If you make it a priority, you can fit anything into a busy schedule." Craig is a busy businessman and has three grade school aged children and still finds time to exercise at least three days per week. In late summer 2003, he was doing a bench press and thought he injured his chest muscle. Turns out it was a cancerous tumor, a sarcoma in his chest muscle. The doctors told him that if he wouldn't have been strength training, he probably wouldn't have found it in time, and it would have spread too fast to save him. He sees exercise as such an incredible blessing, not only for its daily benefits, but also for essentially saving his life.

How does this fit into prioritizing? Craig had to have his left shoulder reconstructed, which meant removing his pectoralis major (chest) muscle in the process and using his latissimus dorsi (back) muscle to replace it, which left him with several limitations in that shoulder. He did, however, have a much higher success rate after his surgery due to all of the strength training he had performed for the past twenty years. Strength training not only gave the doctors more muscle to work with, but Craig also recovered more quickly, because strength training taught his body how to recover more efficiently.

Many people would accept their fate and probably not exercise that part of their body again. But what did Craig do? He *figured out a way to use his left shoulder in as many ways as he safely could.* He told me stories of the different things he tried that worked and that didn't work, and now he has a pretty good idea of what he can and cannot do. Strength training remains a high priority in his life. This goes to show that if exercise is a big enough priority, *you can and will figure out a way* to get it in and get it done, regardless of any limitations you may have, physically or mentally.

Figure out where exercise falls on your priority list

Some know what their priorities are in life while others are spread so thin they see everything as a priority. Things need to be prioritized one way or another in order to get some type of balance back, especially when it comes to your health. If I were to ask you to list your top priorities in your life, your list would probably include the following: entertainment, faith, family, fitness/health, friends, and job/money. The question to ask yourself is: "Do my daily actions match my truest priorities?" As Gandhi stated, "Actions express priorities." Having certain internal priorities and living your life in a totally different way is a low level form of insanity. Unfortunately, many are unaware they are even doing it. All they know is that deep down they are unhappy.

When figuring out where exercise falls on your priority list, keep it in perspective. Is there really anything more valuable to us while we are on this earth than our bodies and our health? Truly look at how your health affects all other aspects of your life before you place it on your priority list. Perhaps you can look at how well you are taking care of yourself versus your car, your home, or other things in your life. Our bodies are the only things that will be with us until the day we die, so I would say that it would be a good idea to prioritize *your* health before these other things that will most likely only last a fraction of your life. What greater priority do you have than to yourself and your health?

If I were to ask you: "Would you take millions of dollars and your ultimate job if it came with a lifetime of health problems?" or "Would you rather be able to enjoy your family being in good health?" most people would give up almost anything to get their health back if they lost it. The problem is that most people wait until the health problem arises to do anything. The main thing is you figure out where your health is on your priority list, understand that exercise is a major part of your health, and begin to live your life according to your priorities and what really matters to you. Too many people would rather spend an extra hour at work trying to get that promotion or going to that party they feel they have to go to than spend the time exercising for their health.

What bites you the hardest? Is it not getting further in your career or not making more money? Is it having a major health problem? Is it walking around every day with the physical and mental burden of the weight you wish would come off, or the pain you are in from being inactive? Money will always be available to earn. If I asked your family members if they would mind if you took a little time away from them each day for your health, as a rule, I bet they *wouldn't* mind and would probably be cheering you on. How would you respond if a family member came to you and asked you that question? Now there is a perspective. Lose your fitness, lose your wellness, and it may never come back. You can't just go buy it in a store (even though a lot of people think you can through surgery and drugs).

I worked with an eighty-four-year-old man who had had a severe stroke. He worked hard for the same company for twenty-five years and loved it, but I bet he would have given it all up to be able to walk right and talk right again. I worked with him on prioritizing recovering from his stroke like he prioritized his job. I know he will improve if he takes this attitude. You may have to treat exercise like another job if you have a great work ethic in your career. Your pay is your health and vitality.

Using your priority list

How do you use your priority list? First of all, you read it every day to remind yourself of where things lie for you and that you intend to live your life more according to this list. You then plan your day or week according to your priorities. This list may shift around as life happens, but keep this list close by. Most people plan their work schedules and family events, then if there is time left over in their busy schedules, they might put in time to exercise or spend time for their faith while their list of what is truly important to them is often inverted to how they are planning their lives (if they are planning them at all).

The ForeverFit plan: As you plan your week, ask yourself, "When am I going to . . . ?" Then fill in the blank with each item on your list in the order of importance. Obviously, a large chunk of your schedule may already be predetermined, but fill in your schedule around these chunks with the top part of your list and work your way down. For instance, faith and health are my top two, because I know without those two as a foundation, the rest of my life suffers. So when I am looking at my week, I ask where I can spend time each day on each item. Since I already know that basically from 6:00a.m. to 8:00p.m. I am committed to work or family so I know the only time to get my faith and exercise in is early in the morning before everyone gets up, or I won't get it in and my work and family life will suffer much more in the long run, and for what—extra sleep?

A powerful way of prioritizing

Attaching a monetary value to your exercise by hiring a personal trainer is a very powerful way of prioritizing, especially if you can barely afford it. By doing this, you are telling yourself your fitness and health are important enough to you to make a financial commitment. This also automatically prioritizes this appointment in your day. If you hire a trainer, make sure they have a strict cancellation policy they stick to. Why? I have learned the hard way that if I am not strict on this with my clients and don't charge people for canceling within a certain time period, they will cancel for a much lesser reason than if I charged them every time. There are always certain things you have no control over, which is understood. However, you need to have something to get you to think about how important this other thing you have to do really is relative to your exercise session. Discuss with your trainer what things should be cancellable reasons before you begin working together.

Another way of putting a monetary value to exercise is by giving to someone you trust—and who will hold you to it—a check at the beginning of each week for an amount that would hurt to part with. You can give that person your commitment to the number of workouts you will do that week. Each workout could be worth a portion of the total amount, or you could make each workout worth the whole amount, whichever will motivate you more. I have done this with clients who were having a hard time doing their workouts outside of working with me, and it works. If exercise was as important to you as it is for FF people, you would never lose that money. Don't feel that would motivate you? What if the check was $1,000? Feel like you could just cancel the check if you needed to? Try cash. Imagine giving your personal trainer or accountability partner $1,000 cash and telling them to keep it if you don't do your workouts that week. Motivated yet? If you feel you wouldn't want to try this technique, you need to truly ask yourself where exercise is on your priority list. If it is high enough, this will be a piece of cake. Pay yourself a portion of this money each week that you succeed. Use it for whatever you want or save it up to get a gym membership, some home exercise equipment, to hire a trainer, or go on a trip.

Priority shifting

Your priorities may shift day-to-day, or week-to-week, so be okay with that. If you have times that other things just have to come first, do what you have to do now and get your priorities back in line ASAP. (You will see this lessen over time if you truly prioritize and take proper perspective.) Tamara (FF 25) says people and relationships can trump exercise. At the time of her interview, her seven-year-old had the flu so she immediately cleared her calendar for the next two days. She claims, "Fortunately, most of my relationships are strengthened because of exercise, and many of my friendships have been formed through exercise." She even met her fiancé when he came to one of her group fitness classes.

If it is a family emergency such as sick children, be there for the family or the kids, tend to them, and be okay with missing a few workouts. Although, who says you can't exercise at home while they are sleeping? I have had sick kids, and I know that when they are sick, they often sleep a lot.

A good idea is to set a time limit on any distraction if you feel it absolutely needs to be done, and stick to that time limit. A better idea yet is to just go exercise, and while doing so, be thinking about how you are going to accomplish this task in an efficient manner. Especially if you are doing cardiovascular exercise and getting the endorphins going, you will often have ideas come to you that you never knew were there. You will also be much more productive when you go back to your task.

If your priorities shift for much more than a week, however, take a good look at what long-term effects this shift will have on you and your health. You are stuck with you for the long haul so don't neglect you. If you aren't prioritizing you, catch yourself and shift your priorities. If you don't, you are a short time away from forgetting the benefits you were feeling from exercise. Typically, you will feel worse for maybe a week or two, but this eventually fades, becomes your new normal, and you begin to tell yourself "I really don't feel that bad from not working out," which, as you could imagine, makes it all the harder to get back on track. This is another big reason why reading your priority list is so important. It helps keep your priorities straight. Having your Morning Meeting with yourself, or exercising first thing, helps you set your priorities right away so you can spend the rest of your day taking care of your other priorities without feeling like you left yourself out of the mix.

When to work out

People have asked me "When is the best time of day to work out?" This question typically stems from reading an article stating that if you work out at a certain time of day, you will burn more calories or lose more weight. The only thing that burns more calories in a given time frame is one thing—*working harder.* That's it. My answer to that question is twofold: Work out at the earliest time in your day when you have the most energy.

If you have a relatively easy time getting up in the morning, get up a half-hour or hour earlier and hit the gym first, before work.

Can't stand mornings? My first suggestion is to try it anyway for six months and see how much better your mornings become. Cathy (FF 5), Mary (FF 27), and many other ForeverFit folks have had to turn themselves into morning people. Not being a morning person is just one of those beliefs that can be changed if you are willing to believe it can change.

The longer you go into your day, the more that can come up to distract you. Karyn (FF 11), formerly Miss Minnesota, says, "I love to wake up early and exercise before my day starts. If I wait to do it later in the day, conflicts often arise." You can lose your sense of priority pretty quickly when those around you do not have the same goals as you. Whenever you choose to exercise is fine; just think of this appointment to exercise as the most important appointment of your day (after your Morning Meeting), because it just may be. If you are not ready for that big of a leap into the earlier morning hours, then your workout needs to be your first appointment after work, if you cannot do it on your lunch hour. No running errands. No going home for a minute, unless it is to grab your gym bag. There is too much that can distract you, like your recliner, e-mail, a load of laundry, and dirty dishes in the sink. So, if you work out at home, it is straight to the workout area. If the kids have a lot to tell you, let them tell you after your workout when you can give them your full attention. If you get into other things first, the next thing you know it is late, you are tired, and even if you go to the gym, your workout isn't what it could have been (although any workout is better than no workout at all).

Notice I said work out when you have the *most* energy, most meaning more, usually. If your only two options are before or after work, try both ways. Give before and after work exercise sessions a consistent effort for a few weeks and check out two things: how well the exercise session went energy wise, and how your days went each way. When you work out early, do you drag through your day or do you have more energy? Is it nice to have it out of the way, or do you think all day about how early you got up? When you work out after work, are you ready to work out the stress from your day or are you dreading it all day long. Once again, pick your perspective. Doing these each for a few consecutive weeks can give you an idea of which works best for you. If there isn't a major difference, exercise first thing in the morning.

It is okay and often more beneficial to split your workouts in half. You could exercise twenty minutes in the morning and twenty minutes at lunch or first thing after work. This can often seem less daunting when you split an exercise session up this way. You can also put your full energy into that twenty minutes since you know the workout isn't that long. You can then see when you get the best workouts, and may be surprised to see that you enjoy splitting them up this way. If so, keep it up!

Emotions and priorities

Ah, our wonderful emotions! Those weightless, formless things that can control so many of our actions. As you read, learn, and relearn the concepts in this book, you may say to yourself, "This is all fine and dandy, but what happens when my emotions get the best of me, and I make the wrong decisions because of them? What can I do about this?"

My friend and client Kim has a PhD, is a licensed psychologist, and specializes in treating individuals with eating disorders. She gave me the background on the logical and emotional parts of the brain, why our emotions can get the best of us, and what to do to help this.

Kim explained to me how information first enters our brains through the emotional center before it hits the logic center. This becomes a problem when our emotions are high, as the information can get stuck in the emotional center, which can make it very difficult for us to think through situations with logic. We therefore react due to these emotions, which doesn't always yield the results we desire. I like to call this "emotional sabotage."

One thing Kim says you can do to help with this emotional sabotage is to first look at what unhealthy actions typically take place when your emotions are getting the best of you. Then you can take steps to choose other responses to your emotional distress.

For example, if your first response to emotional distress is to head to the pantry, liquor cabinet, or to zone out to television, you can use the fact that you are heading this direction to stop yourself and check in on your emotions. If you sense you are in a high state of emotional distress, you can then use other things to calm down your emotional center. These can be things such as play music that calms your mind and lifts your spirits, any form of exercise, or engage in activities such as cleaning or calling a friend. This will give your emotions a chance to calm down so you can think through the situation with logic.

One of the biggest challenges is compliance. Kim said, "Keeping the goal of being more aware and responding differently to emotional distress high on your priority list is critical." She also said to keep in mind what you *will do* when under emotional distress instead of focusing on all the things you won't do.

Priorities trump emotions

So, why did I put emotions in the Power of Priority chapter? First of all, it would be a good idea to put reacting differently to stress high on your priority list. Secondly, if becoming ForeverFit is a big enough priority for you, your emotions will not have nearly the influence on you as you may think.

I had an interesting conversation about this very subject with one of my clients recently. During this conversation, I asked her how often her emotions made her leave work in the middle of the day. She said never. I then asked, "Why is that?" To which she replied "Because I can't," which is code for "Work is too important to me to let my emotions control my actions." Looking at emotions this way shows us our emotions may only control our actions if the thing they are controlling isn't important enough to us. With work, we can see an immediate consequence of leaving (getting written up or fired), but when skipping exercise, we may not see the consequence for months to years, which also makes it easier for our emotions to trump exercise. If becoming ForeverFit is as important as your work, the emotion excuse will be highly diminished.

Have you ever let your emotions get the best of you with a friend or relative, and during that time someone knocked on the door or came into the room and you instantly switched to a nicer attitude?

What happened? Your need to appear as a nice person superseded your emotions. The key is to notice (or become aware) when your emotions are getting the best of you, and create new patterns or responses to your emotional distress. Doing so can give you enough time for your emotions to settle down so you can logically figure out a solution to your issue. Will it work every time? Maybe not, but the more you practice catching yourself, the better you will get and the more it will work. Repeat a new pattern *a lot* until it becomes the normal response to distress.

This concept is so important when it comes to becoming ForeverFit. The concepts in this book are sound and very helpful. However, if you *choose* to let your emotions control your actions, simply knowing these concepts isn't going to be enough at certain times. Becoming ForeverFit has to be a top priority. If it is, you won't let your emotions get the best of you. Don't worry about having emotions. They will always be there and serve you in many ways. Just know what to do with them when they are leading you down the wrong path, and understand that making decisions based on them is generally not a good idea.

Keeping exercise in the right spot on your priority list is a very powerful step for becoming ForeverFit. Just like all new healthy habits, you must practice prioritizing long enough for it to become normal in your life. Figure out where exercise and health lie on the priority list in your mind and be sure your daily actions follow this list.

Applying the power of priorities to your ForeverFit goal

1. Figure out where exercise and health truly lie on your priority list.
2. Plan your week according to this list.
3. Start planning exercise before other things that take you away from it.
4. Know that emotions will more easily get the best of you if exercise isn't a big enough priority.

CHAPTER 5

The Power of Proper Questions

"Successful people ask better questions, and as a
result, get better answers."
Tony Robbins

The above quote lead me to ask myself a question that ultimately helped create this entire chapter. I asked myself, "If this is true, what questions could people ask themselves to help them be successful at becoming ForeverFit?

Asking this question instantly revealed to me the power of asking yourself a proper question. As soon as I asked myself this question, guess what? I received all kinds of answers, and now you will benefit from them.

When I asked myself this question, it is important to note that I received exactly what I asked for. When I asked what questions you should ask to succeed at becoming ForeverFit, I didn't get answers about failing, or answers about relationships, or answers about business. All answers I received related directly to what I asked.

This concept is important as you read the proper questions to help you become ForeverFit. Be aware that whatever questions you ask, you will get a direct answer to.

Get your answers

I once heard if something is told to you, it may be true, but if you discover it for yourself, it *has* to be true. Why is this so important? It is important because if you truly want to become ForeverFit, you must discover the truth within yourself rather than taking my or anyone else's word for it. This is done by asking yourself proper questions and finding your own answers.

The following is a list of ten proper questions that you can ask yourself daily at your Morning Meeting. They will not only tremendously help you begin your day in a positive way, but will become truths for you because you will receive the answers yourself. These truths will then influence your daily actions. This list is not an absolute, so I included a question at the end to help you discover more questions that you may need to help you.

1. How can I be more consistent in exercise? in my Morning Meeting?
2. What can I learn from (enter your mistake, setback, or victory here)?
3. How can I naturally increase my energy so that I can get my exercise in? What things give me a lot of natural energy?
4. What joys do I desire to get from exercise?
5. How can I make time for myself to exercise today and every day?
6. How will exercise benefit all other areas of my life?
7. What is the number one joy-based reason for me to exercise today?
8. How can I make exercise more fun for me?
9. Why is becoming ForeverFit so important to me?
10. What other empowering questions could I ask myself to help me become ForeverFit?

I have pulled some of the questions from other chapters so that you pay close attention to all questions that appear in ForeverFitU and understand their value.

What do you want?

Jesus said, "Ask, and it will be given to you." (Luke 11:9, ESV) What will be given? Well, first of all, answers to what you ask! From your answers, it is your job to take action on the answers you are given. For example, if you ask "How can I naturally increase my energy?" and an answer you receive is, "Eat more fruits and vegetables" you need to eat more fruits and vegetables and stop eating junk food. Be sure to have your actions follow your answers and then they will become truths for you. You can also create a proper follow-up question from your answer. In this example, you might ask, "How can I get myself to eat more fruits and vegetables?" or "What fruits and vegetables would I like to add to my daily nutrition plan?" Then do it!

Sometimes what will be given to you from your questions will be a revelation; something you never realized that you had in you or needed to do. Other times, you may have known the answer, but simply did not apply it. Discovering this for yourself is very powerful. Use these new insights to give you the power and permission to change and become ForeverFit. Keep them in your Morning Meeting to remind you of your discoveries.

Asking questions "as if"

Ask yourself questions "as if" you know you are going to do it. "How am I going to make time to work out today and everyday?" is good. However, this still leaves a little leeway for not finding the time to work out. Better questions are: "When am I going to work out today?" and "What am I going to do in my work out today?" If you are like Karen (FF 38) you could ask, "What time works best today?" These questions are basically telling yourself that you are going to exercise today and it is just a matter of when you are going to do it and what you will be doing when you get there. This leaves no way out in your mind.

End frustration

If you are having a tough time finding the proper questions, ask yourself, "What am I frustrated with right now?" or "What am I upset about right now?" Then, take these answers to discover more proper questions. For example, if you are frustrated with your job and you feel it is sucking the life out of you so much so that you have no energy left to exercise, you might ask, "How can I make my job less stressful?" or "What can I do to enjoy my job more?" or "What other work could I be doing that would provide more enjoyment?"

I have discovered that too often it is the things outside of exercise that are pulling people away from exercising. Therefore, you may have to ask some proper questions about other areas of your life to help you have the time and energy to exercise. Asking questions such as "What areas of my life are pulling me away from exercise?" and "What positive things can I do in these areas to get some balance back?" will help you to ease frustration and allow you to solve your problems your own way. This can dramatically help you get that much needed time and energy you will need to exercise.

Begin asking yourself the proper questions that will give you the proper answers in order to help you take the actions to become ForeverFit.

Applying proper questions to your ForeverFit goal:

1. Ask yourself proper questions if you wish to get proper answers.
2. Include a list of proper questions in your Morning Meeting that will aid you in becoming ForeverFit.
3. Be sure your actions match your answers.
4. Look at other areas of your life that need positive change in order to help you find the time and energy needed to exercise.

CHAPTER 6

The Power of Pictures

**"If you hold a picture in your mind of what you would like to
do or become long enough, it will come true."
Dr. Wayne Dyer**

**"For as he thinketh in his heart, so is he."
Proverbs 23:7 (KJV)**

Your brain works in pictures, not words. In other words, if I were
to ask you to visualize an elephant, you wouldn't picture in your
mind the letters E-L-E-P-H-A-N-T. Instead, your brain sees the
actual animal. Your brain also cannot see the negative or opposite
of something. If I say, "Don't see an elephant," what do you see? You
see exactly what I asked you not to see, an elephant. I was taught in
golf that if there is water on my left and I say to myself, "Don't hit it
left," or "Don't hit it in the water," my brain can only see me hitting it
left, and more often than not, my shot goes into the water. My actions
followed the picture that was in my mind's eye.

This is a very powerful idea, especially when it comes to eating.
For example, many of us say to ourselves we are not going to eat junk
food, while our brain cannot see "not eating junk food" and, like the
elephant and golf example, only sees us eating junk food. Shifting
your mental pictures onto what you intend to do such as, "I intend
to eat five servings of fruits and vegetables per day," is something
your mind can see.

Focus long and hard enough on what you want to do or become and those that you don't will slowly just fade away. They won't have to be stopped. The same goes for losing weight. Your brain cannot see you losing weight, since losing weight is essentially wanting *not* to be at the weight you are at, which your mind actually sees as you wanting *to* be the weight you are at. A much better idea is to see yourself at the weight you would like to be, since your mind can see this. This minor shift can yield major long-term results. Practice seeing yourself at your ideal weight and make sure your daily actions match this picture. As your actions change, this picture will be burned deep into your being, and you will soon become this picture.

Watch out for the word "try"

Saying the words "I will *try* to workout more" is basically sending your mind the picture that you won't. The word try is self-defeating in your mind's eye. If I were to ask you to *try* to pick a pencil off the floor, what does your mind see? It will see you bending over to pick it up, but not doing it. As a matter of fact, you wouldn't even hear someone say, "Can you *try* to pick up that pencil for me?" That is, unless they had a bad back. Instead, you would hear, "Can you pick up that pencil for me?" The word try is used for things you think you may not accomplish, and starting any task with even a smidgeon of doubt as to whether you will complete it is setting yourself up for failure. If that is the case in picking up a pencil, what happens in your mind's eye if you use the word try when wanting to add a healthy habit such as exercise to your life? Stay away from the word try. Catch yourself when you use it and rephrase the statement immediately without it.

Pictures and your daily actions

The quote at the beginning of this chapter states "If you hold a picture in your mind long enough of what you would like to do or become, it will eventually come true." The problem with this law is that it isn't as well known or accepted, simply because most haven't believed in it enough to try it to see if it will come true in their lives.

The reason it comes true is your actions will change as a result of what you see in your mind's eye.

Wayne Gretzky, arguably the greatest hockey player who ever lived, used to have pictures of hockey greats holding the Stanley Cup taped up in the locker room. He and his teammates would visualize doing the same thousands of times. Wayne Gretzky won four Stanley Cups in his career.

Jim Carrey wrote himself a check for ten million dollars, dated five years after he wrote it. In the memo portion of the check he wrote, "for services rendered." He carried this check with him in his wallet so that every time he would see it he could envision earning this money. He not only earned this ten million dollar check within that five-year time frame, less than a decade later he was earning 20 million dollars per film.

Create a feeling with the picture

Both Wayne Gretzky and Jim Carrey visualized what it would feel like if they already had what they were visualizing then and there. It is crucial that you do the same when visualizing becoming ForeverFit.

The pictures you create will have limiting power if they do not have a feeling associated with them. For instance, if you can see yourself at your ideal weight but do not truly feel you will ever be there, you will not have a corresponding feeling with this picture and, therefore, won't act as if you are on your way to it. Close your eyes for a moment and imagine what it would feel like to be at your ideal weight. By the way, your ideal weight is yours, not what some height and weight chart says. Really see it and feel what it would be like if you were that weight *now*. How much more confident would you be? What kind of clothes would you wear in the summertime? What other aspects of your life would dramatically change? See these situations and feel the pictures. From this moment on, live your life as if you are already your ideal weight and are ForeverFit *now*. Let the number that represents your ideal weight remind you to feel these feelings. Live from this feeling and watch how much more energy you have and how much faster you get to your ideal weight.

The wastes that are worry and guilt

No one can deny we all have an imagination. If I asked you to imagine yourself being an astronaut, you could do it. So the question isn't whether you have an imagination, but what you are doing with it. Many people's imaginations are used in destructive, rather than constructive ways. Instead of imagining themselves being successful at whatever they are doing, they spend their imagination on worry and guilt, which are both illusions. Neither is in the now. Worry is nothing but a waste of imagination. It is an illusion of all of the scenarios that might happen and very rarely do.

The biggest problem with worry is the energy it wastes. I heard a great saying once that deserves to be read slowly: "It makes no sense to worry about the things you have no control over, because if you have no control over it, it makes no sense to worry about it. It also makes no sense to worry about the things you have control over, because if you have control over it, it makes no sense to worry about it." Doesn't that cover everything? This is like the serenity prayer: "God grant me the serenity to accept the things I cannot change, the courage to change the things I can, and the wisdom to know the difference."

The bottom line is that you can worry as hard as you want, and it will never solve a problem or change the future. All you have are the decisions you make moment to moment. Don't worry about the fact that you missed a workout or two. Instead, plan your next day to make sure you get it in. Don't worry about what weight you are or that it isn't coming off fast enough. Keep your mind's eye on where you want to be and with consistent effort you will be there.

Guilt is a waste of energy at the opposite end of the time spectrum. Rather than using your imagination to help the future, you spend it regretting the past, which is nothing you can do anything about. If you had a rewind button, that would be great. But you don't. So guilt makes no sense. Instead, as I mentioned before, use your past challenges to help your future by learning from them. Replaying guilty memories in your mind will only waste present moments by zapping your energy and leave you lacking empowerment.

Don't feel guilty about missing a workout. Instead, learn why you missed it. If it is a reason you can control, ask yourself, "What can I do for next time to be sure I get my exercise in?" If it was something you couldn't control, gently remind yourself of this and move on. Trust me; it won't be the last time something out of your control comes up in your lifetime.

What do you think might happen if you began using your present moment energy to see yourself as an avid exerciser, a walker or a runner, a regular aerobics class participant, or a strong, confident person in the weight room? Do you think this would at least get you further along the path to becoming ForeverFit? Understand that anything that is working negatively in you can work even more positively for you if you practice it long enough.

The issue isn't whether you ever worry or feel guilty, but how much attention you place on it. When you notice these feelings, catch yourself and begin to shift your focus to more productive images. It is obviously easier to see these images of you exercising or how you feel after a good workout if you have already experienced them, which the FFs have a lot. Their images of being avid exercisers aren't even conscious thoughts they have to imagine. When you already are ForeverFit, it makes the images of you being a confident, consistent exerciser more automatic. Even if you haven't experienced them yet, carry any image you want with you. Your mind can't tell the difference, anyway. Just as you can see yourself being an astronaut even though you have never been to space, you can see yourself as a fit, lean, confident, avid exerciser if you take the time. Do as Jim Carrey did and *create* a vision if you have to. If you feel worrisome and guilty, you will get the results they bring. On the other hand, if you practice positive images, you will get the results they bring. It is your choice.

Making visualization work for you

If you feel this visualization stuff may work for some but won't work for you, I have a question for you: What picture do you have in your mind of visualization and positive imagery working for you? If you see it not working for you, you will see that it certainly won't work for you. Visualizing visualization working for you should be the first thing to work on. Just for fun, begin by entertaining the idea of visualization working for you. See yourself visualizing things and having them come true in your life. What do you have to lose? What pictures are you holding onto? What Mom and Dad said to you as a child? The way your siblings or friends treated you? The way a teacher or coach treated you? If you continue to see yourself the way you are versus the way you want to be, you will continue the actions that will keep you the way you are. Every action is preceded by a thought, and every thought is a picture. It is that simple. Positive imagery is one of many elite athletes' biggest assets. Seeing the desired results first is what most athletes do who are at the top of their game.

Pictures and weight loss

If you are trying to lose weight or change your body shape, it is a great idea not to look at yourself in the mirror fully or partially naked. Think about what this does to the pictures in your mind. You are burning the current image of yourself right into your brain and you will continue to act upon this image instead of the one you intend to be. Instead, have pictures of yourself when you were the size you want to be on your fridge, in your car, wherever you will see them and say to yourself, "This is who I am." An even more powerful idea would be to ask yourself the question, "What can I do today to begin to look more like myself in this picture?"

You may be saying you do not have a picture because you have never been small. Looking back at the Wayne Gretzky and Jim Carrey examples earlier in this chapter, does this even matter? The key is to hold onto that vision and carry it with you everywhere you go. Creating this vision internally is even more powerful because it will always be with you, rather than a picture you can only see when you look at it.

You could also do what my wife's friend did. She actually took a picture of herself in her swimsuit. Then she cut out muscles on her arms and gave herself a smaller waist and thighs. She posted this picture on her fridge and another copy of it onto her computer to remind her of what she desired to look like.

Developing imagination

You who may be thinking, "I just don't have a good imagination," or "I'm too left brained"; for you, I have just one question that was posed to me in a book entitled *Fanning The Creative Spirit*: Were you ever a child? If your answer is yes, then you have an imagination! It is just covered up by your ego, or the life role you are playing, especially being an adult and all of the things that go along with being mature. This book explains how you can tap into the imagination part of yourself again if you want to. It will just take a little practice (it is fun practice, by the way).

Fanning The Creative Spirit was written by two toy inventors who are masters of simplifying creativity and helping you use that part of your brain that you may not have used for quite some time. It has helped me dramatically in personal training by keeping me creative with programming and helping me think outside the box. It is a great resource to use to help you increase your imagination skills. It also makes you feel like a kid again, which we all could use a bit more of.

Reality versus fantasy

When your mind comes in contact with certain sights, sounds, tastes, and smells that remind you of something in your past, it can give you an emotional response as if it is here now. Have you ever had a song come on that reminded you of a certain good time in your life and you immediately became happy or got goose bumps? How about a certain smell? Maybe a certain perfume reminded you of a high school sweetheart, and all of those teenage emotions came rushing back. I had a client practically burst into tears when an Elvis song came on that reminded her of a loved one who passed away years ago. How did this happen? Her brain thought it was actually occurring.

The key is truly, sincerely telling yourself that being ForeverFit is who you are, seeing it in your mind's eye vividly enough that you generate the corresponding feeling. Visualize it long enough, hold onto the feeling, and your actions will follow. Results are not far behind. I have seen it happen time and time again in my own life.

I used to be the one of the most pessimistic people I knew. I, of course, called myself a realist. After learning I had the ability to choose the pictures I put in my mind and changed my thought patterns long enough, I now live in a totally different and wonderful world that changes for the better all the time, both internally and externally. Do I have down times? Sure. But they are becoming less and less frequent.

See yourself at your ideal, healthy weight. *See* yourself walking into a gym with confidence. *See* yourself enjoying exercise. *See* yourself enjoying healthy food with your family. *See* it over and over! One day you will do it, and it won't seem nearly as scary or difficult. Will all fear be gone? Maybe not, but I guarantee that if you truly and sincerely *see* these things, there will be much less fear. Internally *see* the fat melting off your body when exercising. *See* your heart, muscles, and bones getting stronger. After all, they are! Mary (FF 19) still visualizes her muscles stretching and getting stronger as she exercises.

Each time you see and feel something internally and it comes true, use it to help develop your internal knowing that visualization works. If it doesn't happen right away, it doesn't matter. Keep seeing the right things long enough for it to happen. Every member of the Australian World Cup sailing team visualized every move of the race daily, and they won. What might this do for you?

Other examples of the power of pictures

In *A Second Helping of Chicken Soup for the Soul* there is a great story about a serviceman who was an average golfer who shot in the 90s regularly. When Major James Nesmith became a prisoner of war in North Vietnam, he was held in a cage for seven years. To keep himself sane, he began to play golf in his mind. He would not only visualize the actual course he was playing, every step he was taking, every color and smell, the weather, but he would also see himself making a perfect swing and hitting perfect shots. Round after round he would pass time playing mental golf. When he got out of prison he went out golfing, and without having touched a club in seven years, shot seventy-four, which would be an *amazing* improvement if you *physically* practiced every day for seven years.

Susan Peters' story is another prime example of the power of pictures. She saw herself walking from day one. She sees herself driving again and riding her horses, which I believe she will accomplish. What can stop her? Only her decision to change the pictures she is holding onto. She also has the benefit of seeing her vision of walking actually coming true. But what if she doesn't ride her horses again? What if her physical limitations are just too much? Does that really matter? No. What matters is that holding onto these pictures changes her day-to-day actions for the better.

Do your Morning Meeting, read all of the inspirational things to start your day, write down your intentions, and read them to empower yourself. If you still *see* yourself as a failure, overweight, lazy, or anything negative, your actions will be severely challenged and limited. Fake yourself out for a while if you have to. At least you will live happier as you become ForeverFit.

FF people's pictures

The pictures the people in the FF category hold of themselves inside are so subconscious that they will never be changed, regardless of life's circumstances. They probably don't even realize they have this power within them. Whether or not they used positive pictures to become ForeverFit isn't the point. The point is their pictures are there to stay because they repeated the act of consistent exercise long enough. If I were to ask them how they see themselves as far as fitness goes, I obviously wouldn't hear an answer like "out of shape" or an answer that implies a future state, such as someone who wants to be consistent but isn't yet. They would answer in present tense about being an avid exerciser or being fit. Remember this when it comes to your own pictures. You must see yourself as these people do in present tense, because that is what your brain can see. Make it up if you have to. Jim Carrey did, Wayne Gretzky did, the golfer did, and Susan did, and look what happened to them. The first step is believing that it can and will happen for you.

Applying the Power of Pictures to your ForeverFit goal

1. Pay attention to what pictures you put in your mind on a daily basis.

2. Have a constant picture in your mind of being ForeverFit or having your body look a certain way (if changing your body shape is an end goal) and then take action based upon these pictures. Create this vision if you have to.

3. When you are taking certain actions, ask: "What picture does this send to my mind's eye?" If it doesn't match the picture you want to become, don't do it.

4. Make sure all pictures are in present time even if they may be years away, and that there is a strong, corresponding feeling with the pictures.

The Four Major Shifts

*"Just like the formation of a mountain, long term shifts may
take some time. However, these shifts may also occur in an
instant, like an earthquake."*
Scott Fjelsted

The following chapters are going to dive into some of the specific, major shifts that affect your ability to become ForeverFit. You have the choice of which end of the spectrum to live toward if you wish to become ForeverFit. These shifts will work on the "why" of becoming ForeverFit. As John Kotter, a Harvard Business School professor, stated in *Change or Die*, "Behavior change happens mostly by speaking to people's feelings. In highly successful change efforts, people find ways to help others see the problems or solutions in ways that influence emotions, not just thought." Get to know what you need to do physically and mentally, but make sure your why is in place.

Understand these shifts are not a case of right and wrong. Instead, we will look at the results you get from being at one end versus the other. Simply begin to shift to the end that makes most sense for you in the long run, which is the end that ForeverFit people tend to use. Notice I say in the long run. Using one end will typically help for a while, but that isn't what you want, right? If it seems I am pushing you toward one end, it is only for this reason: I assume you want to be *Forever*Fit. Notice also that I used the word "shift." It isn't as if you need to be 100 percent at one end. Both ends of the spectrum offer some benefit, so use them. You just want to shift more of your energy and attention to the end that will make it easier to become ForeverFit. Keep using ideas from one end; just begin the shift to making the other end the predominant motivator. For instance, many ForeverFit people like Karen (FF 38), Kim (FF 25), and Cathy (FF 5) still use a personal trainer as an external motivator, yet are more motivated by internal reasons like how they feel from exercising, both mentally and physically.

Light some candles

You could also look at each of these two ends less as opposites and more as different levels of energy. As you begin to shift from the lower energy end to the higher, the higher end not only negates the lower, but it converts it into higher energy. This will in turn help keep you going longer. This is like being in a dark room and lighting even a small candle, the darkness (low energy) begins to convert into light (high energy) as long as that candle stays lit. Add more candles, convert more darkness to light.

As you practice these shifts, you will add more candles and make the conversion more permanent, as long as you keep your candles lit by practicing. Just like light and dark have their place, so do these ends of the spectrum. They are all there to help motivate us. The one end will help you for a period of time, while the other end is like what Wayne Dyers called, "An inner candle flame that never flickers," no matter what life throws at you. Work on developing this flame. You will be glad you did.

I will explain which end of the spectrum the FFs tend to migrate toward and what you can do to shift your thinking this way. There is no end to the levels you can reach on these shifts. Reach for the sky!

Applying the four major shifts to your ForeverFit goal

1. Utilize both ends of these spectrums; there is no good or bad, right or wrong.
2. Shift more of your awareness and attention to the end that will best help you become ForeverFit.

CHAPTER 7

Fear to Joy

"Fear kills us more than Death."
George Patton

"There is joy in work. There is no happiness except in the
realization that we have accomplished something."
Henry Ford

Making the first of these four shifts is very powerful simply because it deals directly with your emotions. The two basic ways of becoming motivated and staying that way are joy-based and fear-based. Most people start exercising based on a fear, either from what has already happened or what might happen if they don't start exercising. Losing weight (or fear of getting fat), having a heart attack (or fearing having one), getting cancer or some other disease (or fear of getting one), injury, and potential surgery are all fear-based reasons to begin an exercise program. What is the problem with these fear-based motivators, you may ask? Don't get me wrong; these are all great reasons to begin exercising, but the major issue is that fear tends to fade over time, and, therefore the motivation usually goes right with it.

Remember that tragic day on September 11, 2001? This tragic event evoked fear into our society. Over time people began flying again, choosing not to let their fear rule their actions. In this case, fear fading away was a good thing in many ways. It helped us get back to a sense of normalcy. People started talking about it less and less, and years later it is rarely a topic of conversation. Now, if this event—probably the most horrific thing that has evoked fear on our country's mainland in our generation—has faded in our minds and our actions have shifted back to the way they were, why do we think that having the fear of some fat around our waist or potentially getting some disease is going to keep us motivated?

Fear to joy studies

For a small percentage of people, fear *can* keep them motivated long term. In the article "Change or Die," Dr. Edward Miller, the dean of Johns Hopkins University medical school and CEO of Johns Hopkins University Hospital, stated that many studies have shown that if you look at people two years after they had heart surgery, *90 percent of them have not changed their lifestyles.* He says, "Even though they know they have a very bad disease, and they know they should change their lifestyles, for whatever reason, they can't."

Dr. Dean Ornish, a professor of medicine at the University of California at San Francisco and founder of the Preventative Medicine Research Institute in Sausalito, California, stated in the same article, "Providing health information is important but not always sufficient. We also need to bring in the psychological, emotional, and spiritual dimensions that are so often ignored."

This article also discussed using joy as a motivator. In 1993, Dr. Ornish did a study on 333 patients who had severely clogged arteries who needed heart surgery. After a year of psychology sessions twice weekly, as well as lessons in meditation, yoga, and aerobic exercise, the group was released to work on their own.

In a three-year follow-up study, Dr. Ornish found that *77 percent had stuck with the program of diet and exercise.* Dr. Ornish says that the main reason for change is that motivating people through the fear of dying only lasts a few weeks since these people had the habits they did as a coping mechanism for their emotional states of loneliness or depression. Why would fear of death be a good motivator if you were lonely or depressed? He says that motivating through the joy of living versus the fear of dying is much more effective. "Joy is a more powerful motivator than fear," he stated.

This is great proof of the long lasting power of joy over fear. Joy is a much higher, longer lasting energy, and we all know we need energy to exercise and stay motivated. So why did the 23 percent in this group not stick with it? The most logical conclusion here is they let the fear of recurrence take up too much of their attention and didn't *practice* looking at only the joy in what they were doing. They also probably weren't following much of the contents of this book. Their priorities were misaligned, they lacked perspective, they didn't ask themselves the right questions, the pictures in their minds weren't right, etc. Would you rather have a 10 percent chance of long-term success or 77 percent? Choose joy and increase your odds dramatically.

After September 11, some have chosen to shift their perspectives on terrorism. We know that if we stay afraid, the terrorists win. We go on with our lives and enjoy the things we always have: family, friends, faith, work, and play. We have chosen to live life focusing on the joys of it instead of the fear of what might happen. Those who have not done this continue to live by fear, and that is their choice. This fear prevents some people from flying or going to places where there are large numbers of people. Which one do you think gives you much higher energy on a daily basis? Which one paralyzes you?

Making the fear to joy shift

How do you begin to make this shift? Just like those in the study, we need to begin to eliminate our old reasons for exercising by focusing on newer, higher energy ones. Focusing on the joys of exercise will naturally negate the old fear-based reasons for doing so, and these negative consequences from not exercising will naturally be prevented. Heart attacks will be prevented, you will become your ideal weight, and you will become much happier going into your exercise session. The things you are trying to prevent will be a natural outcome from your daily actions rather than the main reason for exercising.

Tim (FF 7) began exercising at age forty in order to combat high blood pressure and high cholesterol (fear). He also decided it was time to be as healthy as he could for his family and to feel better (joy). Now that he has been consistently exercising for seven years, he sees the other benefits of exercise like the fact that it helps him cope with the stresses of life. Tim woke up before he got a more serious wake-up call. He also has focused more on being healthy for his family than the fear-based reason of what having high blood pressure might do.

Laurie's story

Laurie (FF 25), a forty-something mother of four children, sent me a great e-mail. She has been an avid exerciser her entire adult life. This message from Laurie is a perfect example of not only using joy for motivation, but also using exercise to negate the tough things we all go through in our lives instead of turning to more unhealthy things such as eating comfort foods, drinking alcohol, or taking drugs.

She wrote: "I feel compelled to write about my lifestyle habits because I am so sure they are the reason I feel so good today. I have always lived a healthy lifestyle and feel that eating right, combined with exercise, has been key for me in my life. I left six siblings in Massachusetts when I moved out here to Minnesota twenty-two years ago and we continue to be very close. I miss them all so badly sometimes that I guess I get into a depressed funk and, honestly, the minute I feel this way I get my butt to the gym ASAP. When I leave, I am a new woman. Exercise releases good-feeling hormones in my body. I can be stressed or so sad sometimes, and a good workout is all it takes to cheer me up. No drugs for me, just exercise. I hope this information might help you in your studies of why people do and do not exercise. There are so many people I know on antidepressants, and I just want to tell them to get off them and go exercise. It might not work for everyone, but it sure has worked wonders for me in my life. Another great benefit from exercise is a good night's sleep. I sleep so much better on days I exercise. Be well and live happy."

What a great testament to the power of joy versus fear. Notice you didn't hear one thing about keeping weight off or disease prevention as her motivation to exercise. This isn't to say that those things aren't important to her; it just isn't what she chooses to focus on. Notice also that she says that the *minute* she feels depressed she heads to the gym. This reaction to stress is a great place to get to. What if every time you got stressed out or depressed, the first thing you thought of was exercise to help end it? How powerful would that be? It would turn stress and depression from an excuse to a motivator in an instant. By no means does she or I intend to be a doctor and tell you to get off any medication you are on. Just add exercise to your routine and see what it does for you.

For many like me, this shift from fear-based motivation to joy-based motivation occurs gradually and in stages. I started lifting weights in my teenage years for the sport of Olympic Weightlifting. I was afraid of letting my coaches or big brother down if I didn't show up or work hard, and I was afraid of getting too sore. This eventually shifted into the joy of competition. By my late high school years, I got into vanity, which is essentially fear of what I might look like if I didn't exercise. Over time, my drive to exercise has evolved from injury prevention (fear) and elimination of pain (fear), disease prevention (fear), not gaining weight (fear), into the point now where it is mostly about feeling good (joy) emotionally, mentally, physically, and spiritually, as well as having a healthy body.

Many people don't make it through the fear stage due to lack of knowledge of the power of joy, but I stayed motivated enough through those stages to evolve to the joy stage. I think a big reason is that underlying the vanity in my early years of exercising was the confidence it gave me and how I felt after a good workout. I am blessed these fear-based reasons were not the major motivator.

Feed your joy

The beauty is you can choose to get to the joy stage *right now*, without having to evolve, as I did. It is simply a matter of what you choose to focus on. Focusing on the joys of exercise will delete the fears of what may happen if you don't exercise. Make the decision today to focus on the joys of exercise. Even if it is just one joy, do it. More will come later. If you cannot think of one single joy that might come from exercising, sincerely ask yourself, "What joys could I find about exercise if I had to?" Begin to ignore thoughts of exercise being too hard or taking too long. Remember, however, that just as fear fades if you stop focusing on it, so can joy. Focus is like a muscle. Exercise it and it gets stronger. Fail to use it and it weakens. This will be a major thing to remember as you go through the next chapters on the other shifts to be made.

Focus is a choice; only you may have been choosing (consciously or unconsciously) to focus on the end that has yielded you the results you don't want. I heard a great story that illustrates this point: A father was saying to his son, "I feel I have two wolves living at war inside me. The one is fearful, hateful, and thinks about all of the bad things in my life, while the other is loving, compassionate, and thinks of all of the joys in my life." When the son asked his father which one he thinks will win, his father replied, "Whichever one I feed."

Start feeding your mind joyful reasons for exercising long enough and joy will win. Joy isn't something you will have to look for; joy will become your constant companion as you become ForeverFit.

The one joy we all share

If you still are having a hard time finding any joys about exercise, there is one joy that we all share: the miracles that are our bodies. Although there are many shapes and sizes, the function of our bodies is an absolute miracle, especially when you exercise them. The trillions of cells that need to work simultaneously just to get your muscles to contract, therefore causing you to breathe harder and your heart rate to increase, to adapt to body temperature changes by sweating, to shift blood flow from your organs to your muscles, and to utilize fat, protein, and carbohydrates in the perfect proportion for the given exercise intensity are an absolute miracle. If you were to look at the muscles that work together to simply walk, you would be amazed. If I went into the science behind being able to propel your body in a forward direction, it would blow you away, not to mention it would double the length of this book. All of these things happen without you having to consciously tell yourself anything.

If you are having a hard time finding any joys during the exercise session you are in, simply become more aware of the miracle that is taking place in the present. There are people who do have to think about every step they take, as Susan Peters did at one point. Becoming aware of these things that you highly took for granted can be a great source of joyful energy. Do you think it is hard to exercise now? What if you had to tell yourself to breathe harder or your heart to beat faster as you exercised? The fact that you don't have to do this makes just having to get off your butt and simply move seem a whole lot easier.

Other joys of exercising

So what other joys are there about exercise and becoming ForeverFit? Many, like Tina (FF 21), love the natural high they get from the endorphins. Those like Steve (FF 28) really appreciate the alone time they get each day, while others, like Lora (FF 32), love the social aspect of a health club. Some, like Gwen (FF 20), feel a connection with God when they are fit and healthy. Others, like Craig (FF 23) and Cathy (FF 5), get joy from being sore from an intense workout. Some type-A personalities like Erik (FF 20) get part of their joy from achieving goals. Some, like Mary (FF 27), enjoy the sense of accomplishment from a good workout and simply feeling strong and healthy. Lastly, some, like Karyn (FF 11), love the feeling of self-discipline that consistent exercise brings that they can carry over into other aspects of their lives.

Be here now

One big joy you can experience from exercise, especially intense exercise, is experiencing the now. So much of our mental energy is unfortunately used up thinking about the past and future, while the present moments keep slipping away. Truly experiencing the present moment gives you tons of energy, mainly because the now is all we really have. This is another reason why exercise is energy giving. It is impossible to exercise your hardest and think about all of the stresses in life. This is a big reason to challenge yourself during your workout. When it is too easy, or you are just going through the motions, your mind can wander, often onto the thoughts you really don't want to dwell on.

Use your workout time to practice being in the moment. See what joy and energy it brings. Make your workout your time to do something good for yourself. Don't muck it up with thoughts of anything but how hard you are working, especially if you have had a bad day, week, or month in other areas of your life. It is a good idea to keep cell phones and other things that can interrupt you away from your workout area. Trust me, your problems will all be there waiting for you when you are done exercising.

If you want fitness to be more than just a physical act, make it something you use to escape life for awhile, and learn to be in the moment by working hard. If intense effort isn't your thing, do your best to count every repetition you are doing if it is a strength training day, or count your breaths as you stretch. This has proven to help keep some of my clients in the moment if they are prone to letting their minds wander.

Take up yoga

Gwen (FF 25) has been doing yoga since 1992 and teaching since the year 2000. She once told me that those who take yoga for an extended period of time tend to naturally want to treat their bodies better by exercising more and putting better food into their bodies. Gwen has such a love and passion for yoga. Her passion shines through in the way she teaches. The following is a statement I had Gwen write up for me on what yoga means to her and what it has done for her life. Much of it fits right in with many of the concepts in this book. Like everything written in this book, take something from this that may help you to naturally treat your body with the respect it deserves, for joyful reasons rather than fearful ones. Be open and ask yourself, "How can this help me find joy in exercise, and life for that matter?"

Yoga: how it changed and defined my life

"What started with purely physical intentions produced a profound spiritual and psychological change.

I started practicing yoga because I loved the beauty of the practice. I was a dancer, singer, and performer, and yoga kept me flexible and strong. I liked the way it toned and shaped my body. The practice worked from the outside in. Slowly I delved more deeply into the science of a yogic lifestyle.

The philosophy of yoga rung true for me. The principles slowly seeped into my daily life, and I felt when I lived a more yogic life, I was happier and much more balanced. What is a yogic life? To me, a yogic life is a *clean* life: clean thoughts, relationships, diet, etc. By clean, I mean true. True meaning a life free of self-deception. When rationalization and deception are a part of life, it is impossible to live fully.

Another principle, *ahisma,* or non-violence, is a key component to living a yogic life. Non-violence means not doing any harm. When we eat food that does nothing positive for the body, we do harm. When we do not move our bodies daily, over-eat or under-eat, over-exercise or become lazy, we are doing violence to our own bodies, minds, and spirits. This principle can be applied to all aspects of life. God created the body, earth, sky, and all other living creatures. All should be treated as holy and cared for with respect. We get into trouble when God's creations are abused or taken for granted. We may get away with the abuse for a while, but it eventually does have an effect, if not immediately. Being mindful is the key.

Another key principle in yoga is taking only what you *need.* This is a difficult practice for the Western world, as success is often measured by what we *have* and not *who* we *are.*

I have found that when I rationalize a bad choice, it is all the easier to do it again, creating a pattern. It is okay to make mistakes, but yoga is about seeing the mistake, not judging it, and making a different choice the next time. It is self-love. I have found much joy, peace, and health through practicing the yogic principles to the best of my ability."

Take up yoga. See if it helps you see more of the joy not only in life, but in exercise and eating as well.

Shifting from fear to joy

1. Ask yourself, "What are the joys I find in exercise?"
2. Become aware of when fear-based motivators creep in, and shift back to the joyful reasons you are choosing to exercise.
3. Feed your mind joy.
4. Take up yoga.

CHAPTER 8

External to Internal

"Inspiration is something that tends to capture
you rather than you capture it."
Joan Armatrading

"You cannot help men permanently by doing for
them what they could and should do for themselves."
Abraham Lincoln

As Joan Armatrading's quote states, inspiration grabs you and takes
your actions where you are destined to go. External motivators
constantly have to attempt to take you where you need to go. The
higher the level of inspiration that you reach, the fewer external
forces you need to drive you. When you begin to focus on the joys
of exercise, your internal motivation increases. Although this shift
needs to happen for long-term success, external motivators are always
helpful to have along the way and are sometimes needed during those
tough days when exercise is the last thing you would want to do.

For most FF people, there was an initial need for external
influence to get them on the track to fitness and better health. This
could be in the form of another person, such as a family member or
friend, a coach, a doctor, a movie, a book, or a success story. John (FF
25) had a group of three other guys he worked out with during the
weekdays who gave him tons of encouragement. These relationships
are things that can keep you going, simply for the relationship aspect,

and look at the side benefit you get. For Erik (FF 20), it was his football coaches and teammates.

We claim that many of these external things inspire us, and they do if they put something inside of us that makes us behave differently. Don't let me make you think external motivation is bad or wrong. If it were, I wouldn't be writing this book. I also wouldn't have been a personal fitness trainer for the last decade. Its only problem is that as soon as that external thing goes away, the motivation may go with it. Your trainer quits, moves, or you feel you can't afford it any more (watch your perspective); the movie, book, or CD that once motivated you has lost its luster; the friend or family member who got you going either quit themselves or seems to be at too high a fitness level for you to keep up, etc. As Craig (FF 23), says, "The external things change too much to rely on them."

External motivators have value

There will always be motivators out there, and I would suggest plugging as many inspirational books, CDs, movies, etc. into you as possible as a way of making this shift inward. Eventually, through daily practice, you will begin to develop the knowledge that motivation also lies within you, not just from someone or something outside of you. The more you read about and listen to the ForeverFit people that you want to become like, the more their words will become your own, and your daily fitness habits will soon mimic theirs. Even the suggestions in this book will eventually begin to just flow out of you if you take the time to let them become part of you. Something inside you told you to read this book. This same power inside you wants to help you change.

ForeverFit folks use external motivators, such as music, DVDs, motivational tapes, other workout buddies, exercise classes, and personal trainers just to name a few. What they also have is an internal flame that is there for them when their external motivators aren't present.

One very powerful thing about developing internal motivation is that it is permanent. Once you achieve this internal understanding that the values of exercise in your life are *the way* to live, nothing can stop you. Your focus becomes more automatic. Life circumstances will no longer make you choose unhealthy habits. Instead they will drive you to exercise. Every FF person I interviewed for this book has this *knowing* that exercise virtually always makes them feel better both mentally and physically. No one has to tell them they will feel better when they are done exercising; they already know from experience.

Adding silence and meditation to your Morning Meeting

One of the biggest things you can do to make this shift to inspiration is to make the Morning Meeting with yourself a little longer—say 20 to 30 minutes. This isn't a given number; it may be longer or shorter for you. Read those things you have written about how you intend to be for the first few minutes, and then sit quietly and meditate on them for the next five to twenty minutes. Just sit and breathe, thinking of one or two empowering words of the day such as joy, perspective, energy, and consistency to use as your inner mantra. Do this before the hectic day sets in.

For some, this seems like it would be a waste of time, especially for those wrapped up in our "do" society. Don't feel like you have the time? Why not meditate on these things while exercising? If you are at a health club, put your headphones on, but don't turn on the music. No one will bother you. Some feel that if you aren't doing something, you aren't accomplishing anything. As if working on your mental, spiritual, and physical health isn't accomplishing anything. Quieting the mind is one of the greatest things you can do for yourself. I have been doing it daily now for years and the internal growth it gives is amazing. It is where truth lies, truth being who you really want to be and what you really want to accomplish for all the right reasons. Don't let me give you the wrong idea about doing. I dedicate a whole chapter on it later. You just need to understand the power of doing combined with non-doing.

Lao Tzu said, "Silence is a source of great strength." Mother Teresa said, "We need to find God, and He cannot be found in noise and restlessness. God is the friend of silence." Psalms 46:10 (NIV) says, "Be still and know that I am God." So many people spend their entire lives with the TV and radio on, talking, doing, and we wonder why we don't have the inspiration to do healthy things for ourselves. There is a whole other world inside of you waiting to help you change your life for the better, and it is much easier to get to with silence.

Meditation isn't a religious thing, yet isn't non-religious either. It is connecting to that higher part of yourself that we all have, the part that feels it can do anything. George Kenworthy, senior pastor of Wayzata Evangelical Free Church in Plymouth, Minnesota, wrote in his book *Marriage Makeover*, "Prayer is talking to God, while meditation is becoming silent and letting God talk to you." This can only occur in silence. The more you practice meditation, like anything else you practice, the better at it you become. Through meditation, the higher part of yourself negates your ego, where all of the fear and doubt is, and you become internally motivated.

Since I am not an expert on meditation, I am not going to get into a lecture on the specifics of it. Like all things in life, you won't know how something works until you sincerely use it. Just as I can't justly explain to someone who is sedentary what it feels like to be fit or what it feels like at the end of a workout, I can't explain what it feels like to meditate. You get out of it what you sincerely put into it, and you won't know its benefits without the experience of it. It would be like trying to explain to someone what water was without him or her ever seeing, touching, or tasting it. When you come to a point in your day and you don't want to exercise, you can draw on this meditation experience to get the energy you need to get moving. As a matter of fact, your meditation will eventually flow out of you through positive action. After all, getting started is often the hardest step.

Faith and Fitness

I am very grateful to have been brought up in a family of faith. Growing up, it amazed me how many people at church weren't taking care of their body temples. I would hear things like, "God loves you no matter how you look," and "It's what is on the inside that counts." Although these things may be true, I have found that if I am not taking care of my body, it is *extremely* hard for me to connect to God. This goes back to silence. If your mind is being taken up with thoughts about how fat you are, or how out of shape you are, or how tired you are, connection with divinity becomes extremely difficult. I have found that the better care I take of myself, both physically and mentally, the easier it is to be in silence. The easier it is to be in silence, the easier it is to have energy to exercise. Do you see the pattern? If you would like to grow spiritually, get fit and see how much easier it is to connect with God. Even if growing spiritually is not a goal for you, I bet you wouldn't mind feeling better on a daily basis.

The value of silence

The following is something I wrote one morning at about 3:30a.m. when the world is silent. It does a good job summarizing the value of silence.

Rumi said, 'The morning breeze has secrets to tell you. Do not go back to sleep.' I have found this to be true. Get up before the world does. Take that time of day to discover that deeper, true part of you. Don't read the paper. Don't turn on the TV. Just be in silence with yourself. No thinking about what you have to do today. No thinking about how much or how little sleep you got. Just you and your notes of who you want to be and what you truly want to accomplish, becoming ForeverFit. Throughout your day, you can draw back on this time with yourself when the pressures of life get to you. It is much harder, if not impossible, to do your Morning Meeting when the rest of the family is up or you have ten other things on your mind that you should be doing. Getting up a little earlier can give you this time.

I can tell you from experience that if you give yourself time to get used to it for a consistent amount of time, these early morning hours will be some of the greatest times of insight and inspiration for you. Some of the things you have been struggling with for a long time will be changed internally in an instant. Just make sure it is the morning breeze, not the morning news.

Most FF people have some sense of inspiration, whether they know it or not. This has nothing to do with their faith, although it helps. It has more to do with their internal knowing that what they are doing is right and good for them. This internal knowing supercedes any temporary pain or effort that goes into a workout. Pam (FF 39) calls the pain from exercising a "healthy pain."

Internalizing your goals

One other thing you can do to shift yourself to more internal motivation is to not tell anyone about your goal (except of course your accountability partner) or what you are changing about yourself. This is very powerful because it keeps you focused on what you have to do for yourself versus for others. It also feels like you have this secret you are accomplishing that you will surprise everyone with by getting results.

Having accountability is a great thing to have at first, don't get me wrong. It is a big reason why people have such great success with personal trainers. It is also a big reason why 90 percent of heart patients can't change their lifestyles, but 77 percent of Dr. Ornish's patients could—because he gave them support groups weekly with other individuals in the program, as well as help from dieticians, psychologists, nurses, and yoga and meditation instructors. ("Change or Die," Fast Company, May 2005)

Does this mean you have to go this far and have all of these people in your entourage to become successful? Of course not. This is where a good personal trainer can be a huge help to not only guide you on a proper path, but to be that much needed support system if you do not have a good one to talk to about any struggles you are having and how to work past them. If you want to create more permanent change when you are out on your own, become accountable to yourself as well. We have already discussed one of the best ways to be accountable to yourself and have your own psychology session—your Morning Meeting.

More on accountability

Being accountable to yourself doesn't mean punishing yourself for being bad. It means checking in with yourself to keep you progressing toward becoming ForeverFit. Keep your accountability partner, workout buddies, and fitness classes. Keep your personal trainer if they are providing you value. Have them help you with guiding and motivating you through your fitness regimens, as well as working on the concepts in this book. Just make sure you are doing your part and you will multiply your efforts tenfold. I assure you that all of these people would like nothing more than to see you become ForeverFit and to maximize your efforts during your time away from them. These people can only be with you a limited amount of time. How much are you with yourself? Do the math.

Inside all of us is an internal knowing. This knowing is one that leads us all to the truth of the value of exercise in our lives. It is the part of ourselves that always wants to say a kind word, lend a helping hand. It is the part of us that is true to ourselves about what we truly want in life, rather than instant gratifications, which fade so fast and cost us so much. The only way to get to this part of ourselves is through silence. No techniques needed. Just add silence and thoughts of peace, not about what we have to do in our day, just peace and kindness. Direct this peace and kindness toward yourself, not just to others. If you are constantly thinking thoughts of peace and kindness toward yourself, you will be more likely to treat your body with the respect it deserves. Develop this internal motivation and watch habits naturally change. Aren't you worth it? Remember the wolf story from the fear to joy chapter. Feed this internal motivation.

While developing this internal motivation, it is always good to have a quote (or twenty) to help keep you going. When you come across a quote you find motivates you, internalize it by drilling it into your head every day, and one day connect it straight to your heart. Get here and have a powerful ally. The following are some internal quotes that some FF people say to themselves to keep them going:

- "Life is for the living." Pam (FF 39)
- "Get going . . . you will be done before you know it, and then you will be happy with yourself." Tina (FF 21)
- "I can do this." Cathy (FF 5)
- "Get up and get out. This is for me!" (Suzanne (FF 23)
- "Move and live, sit and rust." Mary (FF 27)
- "Stop whining, no excuses." Karen (FF 38)

Shifting from External to Internal Motivation

1. Keep using your external motivators, such as personal trainers, music, television, social interaction, quotes, etc. that keep you exercising.
2. Meditate daily, in silence, even if it is only for five minutes.
3. Shift to an internal motivation through repetition, putting external motivators deep within you, as well as through your experiences.

CHAPTER 9

Reading to Doing

**"It is no use saying 'We are doing our best.' You have got to
succeed in doing what is necessary."**
Winston Churchill

**"A life making mistakes is not only more honorable, but more
useful than a life spent doing nothing."**
George Bernard Shaw

You may be thinking that the opposite end of doing would be doing
nothing, but I don't need to go that far if you are reading this book.
Instead, I will talk about those who read book after book, but nothing
ever seems to change. They may come up with all kinds of excuses
like not having enough discipline, or having a bad upbringing, or
some other circumstance as to why they never succeed. I heard a
great comment from a mentor of mine years ago. He was talking
about this concept of doing and said he was going to write a book on
how to be successful at anything. There was going to be 300 pages,
299 of which would be blank. One page in the middle of the book
was going to have five simple words:

GET
UP
OFF
YOUR
BUTT!

The funny thing was that this was talking directly to me. This was dealing with selling, something I wasn't too hot at. I would go from book to book, lecture to lecture, yet wouldn't do anything afterward to utilize what I was learning. I kept getting the same results, which was next to nothing. This could easily apply to becoming ForeverFit as well. Was it the lectures' or book writers' fault that I didn't succeed? Of course it wasn't, because many people were successful from using these tools. I didn't succeed because I wasn't doing anything with what I had learned. I had to get up off my butt!

Discipline

I heard a great definition of the word discipline by a very successful businessman named Tim Sales (good last name, huh?). He defined discipline as simply "doing what you need to do long enough until you get the desire you want." That is all it is. All you need to ask yourself is, "Have I reached the place I desire to be (becoming ForeverFit)?" and, if not, you simply keep doing. You continue to do your Morning Meeting. You continue to exercise consistently so that it becomes a more normal part of life. The problem is most people quit before they have reached their desires. They lose focus on why they are doing what they are doing. If you go into a fitness regimen thinking "If I don't get to a certain weight or fitness level by a certain date, I'm going to be upset, or worse yet, quit," you are heading for trouble.

Be sure that your short-range goals don't determine whether you keep going or not. They are simply used as guides along your path. You can use them to see whether what you are doing is working, and if what you are doing isn't, change what you are doing.

Reading

Reading accomplishes education, which is a very important first step. You need reading to get yourself on the right track and keep you there; a map, if you will. If you had a map of the United States and figured out exactly how you were going to drive from Minnesota to California and kept looking at the map over and over until you knew that route like the back of your hand, but never left your living room, how much closer would you be to California? You get the analogy. Yet that is often what many do when it comes to their fitness habits. They gain so much knowledge of what to do but are doing nothing on a daily basis to get to where they want to go.

The FFs and doing

The FF folks do much less reading and much more doing. They know something is better than nothing; any movement is better than none. Yes, many of them keep themselves educated by books, magazines, and fitness professionals, but no matter what, they continue doing. Some of them are almost too extreme at the opposite end and do little or *no* educating, which often leads to overtraining and injury. This is when they often seek out help from a professional. They will do anything to make sure they can continue to exercise.

Read this book and others daily. But most importantly—*start doing*! Go on a walk. Join a gym. Join a community education aerobics, strength, or yoga class. Have a trainer come to your house at first if you have to. Find a workout partner who is more motivated than you. Start small and slow. Those who make small improvements day by day tend to stick with their new habits much better than those who try to do a bunch of new habits all at once, only to get overwhelmed and quit. At least get started. Although starting is often the hardest part, thinking about starting is even harder. Even if you decided to walk to California, you would still get there faster than if you continued to sit and study the map. Have the map in your pocket; just keep walking. In our fast paced, instant gratification society, we want to get there in a Ferrari, or better yet, a Leer jet, if we have the funds. Becoming ForeverFit isn't a race, and California is California, whether you get there in an hour or a year. The whole purpose is to get there, and once you are there, you can choose to stay or not. If it is mid January, you are probably going to stay. Is your fitness lifestyle in a mid-January stage? Start that walk. You will be in a warmer climate before you know it. Want to get there in a Ferrari? *Apply* what is in this book on a *daily* basis and you will!

Successful doers

I had a client who is a very successful salesman. I asked him why he felt he had the success he has had, outselling 90 percent of his company ten to one, yet working half the hours. His secret: he is a doer. Rather than mapping out a perfect strategy of how he was going to get customers, he was out pounding the pavement, talking to them directly. He was at appointments rather than spending all of this time waiting for people to call him back. He also understood the value of how much you learn by doing; learning from disasters and mistakes rather than getting depressed or down about them. You can carry this over in your journey to becoming ForeverFit.

Susan Peters is a doer. Do you think she had a clue how she was going to walk again, yet alone complete a 5k? No one in her condition had ever accomplished that. She just began doing. She sought out the experts. If the one she was with wasn't getting her what she needed, she found another. She just kept on smiling and doing, changing things when needed.

"Do-Do" list

The "do-do" list is a list of things to do *now, today*. Not things that you hope or wish to do, but your now list. Start with something simple, especially if you are just starting out. I encourage people to join a gym simply because of the financial obligation (priority), as well as having a place to go where you can see that you aren't the only crazy person doing this exercise thing. There is also power in the fact that if you have a place to go, it becomes more like an appointment that you have to stick to than if you do it in your home, where there are a thousand other things that always need to be done. Too intimidated to go to a gym or lacking the funds? Start by going on daily walks and buying some cheap in-home equipment such as an exercise ball, resistance bands, and dumbbells. Can't hire a trainer yet? Read a book on exercising at home. Keep this "do-do" list current. It will need to change as your goals do and as your confidence grows.

The mentality of joining a gym

Understand one big thing about going to a gym: If you feel intimidated or are overweight, know that people aren't staring at you. They aren't judging you. If anything, they are thinking how great it is that you are taking a step in the right direction. Most people are so into their own workouts that they hardly notice anything else. I can tell you that from personal experience. Remember, you are there for you, not them. With experience comes confidence, and you only get experience by doing. In his book *What Do You Really Want For Your Children,* Dr. Wayne Dyer stated, "You build self-confidence by doing; not by worrying, thinking about it, talking about it, but by doing." The same goes for reading this book or watching other success stories. These things may inspire you, but nothing will increase your self-confidence more than doing.

I heard a great saying once that you become who you hang around. With this in mind, be careful not to join a gym where everyone seems to be overweight or one that seems like it's not where you want to be, unless you absolutely have to at first to get yourself moving. This environment can leave you in a comfort zone that can keep you from growing. Go to a place full of vibrant, fit people. Don't be intimidated by them; strive to become one of them. Watch what they are doing, and one day you will become them. If you still can't see yourself joining a gym like this, find one that you are comfortable with for now, get fit, and switch when your confidence level grows.

Fear and doing

If you aren't afraid to walk, you can't be afraid to *do.* If you are afraid to take the first step to join a gym but know it is time to do so, *do it afraid!* You will see that it isn't nearly as scary as you thought. As a matter of fact, one of the greatest things you can do to motivate yourself is to do something when you are afraid and get past your fear. It is one of the greatest steps for growth that can create a snowball affect into trying more and more things you never thought you would. You not only get this huge burst of energy from doing it while you're afraid, but you also squash the fear. Use your personal trainer or accountability partner to tell them your fears and take steps to *do it while you're afraid*. Watch the energy you get when you get through it. Use this energy for the next scary thing you undertake. Most people end up regretting the things they don't do much more than the ones they do.

Big talkers

Talking about what you are going to do, especially to those who don't have the same goals as you, does nothing but waste air. As I stated in the last chapter, you lose the power of internalizing your goal when you talk about it a lot. There is nothing wrong with telling an accountability partner, having confidence, or telling someone who asks you, but do more doing than talking. This would be like sitting in your living room for a month, calling everyone you know, and telling them about this trip to California you are going to go on. If you would have just left, you could have called them from the beach. Do your talking after you have become ForeverFit. Tell friends, family, and strangers how great it feels to be there and how you intend to stay. Invite others to visit. Tell them you would be happy to show them the route. Become a source of inspiration. Showing others how to get where you have gone can help spread health and wellness to the world, which is one of the greatest gifts you can give, and it costs you nothing.

I heard a great story that illustrates big talkers. Dr. Wayne Dyer had a patient who was upset because she never learned how to ride a bike. Instead of getting into the deep psychological reasons why she couldn't ride a bike, he decided to get her on a bike, right then and there. He then explained to her that the only reason she couldn't ride a bike is that she had never gotten on one, and once she did and fell on her butt a few times, she would learn. They could have sat there and talked about her past and all of her psychological barriers, but until she was willing to actually take the step of doing, she would never have learned anything. Be willing to make mistakes, to slip and fall. Be willing to get a little off course from time to time. Just get back on course and keep on doing.

Doing and your knowing

One of the most powerful things that doing will accomplish is develop your deep knowing of the rewards of exercise. Once you have this knowing, no person or thing will be able to tell you it isn't true. Every single ForeverFit person I interviewed has this knowing. Any time ideas come from an external source they will always come attached with some type of doubt. Ask ForeverFit people if they have doubt about the benefits of exercise in their lives. What do you think their response would be?

If you became the world's biggest expert on how to ride a bike, but had never actually gotten on one, even you wouldn't have 100 percent confidence on your ability to ride it. Show me a five-year-old who has fallen on his butt a couple dozen times before learning how to ride, and I will show you someone who has developed a knowing. Within a short period of time this lad would have ten times more confidence in being able to ride a bike than an expert who has never actually been on a bike. It is like the experts who said Susan would never walk again. Who do you think has more knowledge of whether it is possible for someone in her situation to walk again? Experience what exercise can do for your life if you do it consistently and long enough. It will become more like a privilege than a chore.

Once you have been doing long enough (exercising, having your Morning Meeting, etc) and have become ForeverFit, you may not be where you would like to be physically. If so, you must change something, either in your exercise or your eating, most likely a combination. In my experience with most ForeverFit people who still aren't at their ideal weights, nutrition is a huge part of the battle. This is where finding a quality nutrition expert can be a big help. You can save a lot of time and frustration by going to someone who can look at what you are currently eating and who can help you change what needs changing. Albert Einstein defined insanity as "doing the same thing over and over again and expecting different results." If you are expecting different results, what you are doing must change.

Shifting from Reading to Doing

1. Keep reading and educating yourself as you become ForeverFit.
2. Keep doing to develop an inner knowledge that will be your solid foundation.
3. If your doing isn't getting you the physical results you desire, seek out a professional to help you change your routine or help you with nutrition.

CHAPTER 10

Short Term to Long Term

"There is no finish line."
Bob Harper

"There are risks and costs to action. But they are far less than
the long range risks of comfortable inaction."
John F. Kennedy

Everything in this book so far has stressed the importance
of shifting more toward thinking long term instead of short
term (I titled it "**Forever**Fit" for a reason). This quote by Bob
Harper, a celebrity fitness trainer and a personal trainer on the
reality show *The Biggest Loser,* is such a great way to look at
exercise. If you practice feeling like there is no finish line, your
whole perspective on what you are doing changes. What do
people do at finish lines? They slow down and eventually stop.
When becoming ForeverFit, there is no stopping. You may veer
off course, but never stop. You must never get to the point of
thinking you have been consistent six months or a year so now
you've got it all down. Never feel like you have it all down now
or that you know all there is to know about fitness or personal
growth. Be willing to learn from everyone. This only occurs
if you are willing to see other people and circumstances as
teachers. If you were to learn everything there is to know, how
boring would that be?

The issues with the short run

Most people start exercising for shorter-term reasons: a vacation where they have to wear a bikini or swimsuit, a wedding, reunion, summertime coming, etc. Many people think this way because of our microwave, drive-through society of now results, eight-minute abs, or twenty-minute, three-days-a-week workouts to look like the people in the infomercials. Even weight loss tends to be a short-term thought process, even if it may have taken twenty years to put that weight on. Once again, these are fine reasons to get on an exercise regimen. Anything that makes you more active is good. But what happens when this short-term event comes and goes? Most go back to their old habits. Sound familiar?

Why think long term?

First of all, as I discussed earlier, there is no finish line. So having a short-term event can end up feeling like a finish line, and you can too easily lose your focus afterward. When thinking long term, you see the next short-term event simply as a stepping stone along the way to becoming ForeverFit. This upcoming event simply gives you a short-term focus to make your training more interesting. Thinking long term makes it much easier to stay on track once the recent event has passed.

Secondly, when you have a bad day, week, or month, you won't get down or discouraged because there is no finish line. These bad times will only be a blip or a bump in your road to long-term success, rather than a time to contemplate whether you are succeeding or failing. I have a client who started a company from scratch and built it into one that employed over one hundred people. He sold it for tens of millions forty-four years later. Do you think he would have had this long-term success if every time he lost a customer or had an employee problem he went to his office and contemplated what he was doing or wallowed in this setback? He just brushed it off and kept on going. He also said that he always had fun (focus on joy). I see people all the time that beat themselves up for a less than perfect week of exercise. Doing this too often is self-sabotage. Brush yourself off. What matters is that you are still making an effort years from now, not whether or not you missed a workout once or twice this week. Don't beat yourself down; build yourself up.

I once heard a client say to herself, "I'm so stupid." I asked her why she thought that, and she told me what she had done. The funny thing is that it was something that I do all the time. So I told her that I do that all the time too and asked her if she thought I was stupid. She said "no," of course. I replied, "Then why would you think you were stupid, if you were simply doing the same thing I was and you don't think I was stupid?" She got the point. Treat yourself like your best friend. If he or she had a bad day or week, you wouldn't tell him or her what a loser or failure he or she was. You would say, "That's okay! Let's get going again." You would tell them you are there for them no matter what. Your self-talk *can* be controlled and used to your advantage. Notice when your self-talk becomes self-defeating, and start to talk to yourself like a friend who has your long-range health in mind. It can help a lot.

Goals

Setting short-term goals is great and often necessary to keep you on track. Having that carrot out there can often keep you going for a while. But unless there are more carrots to put out there right after the one you just got to, you'll start to lose momentum. If you have short-term goals, use them. Put a picture of your vacation destination everywhere you can to remind yourself to eat right and exercise.

It is great to have goals. It is often what can get and keep you going, especially if you have ever used goals for success in other areas of your life. Erik (FF 20) still likes to use things such as upcoming 5ks and trips to set goals and keep himself motivated in the short run, while in the long run he views exercise as "something that will prevent me from becoming immobile and unable to do things." Erik has used goals successfully in his business and sees their value in helping him in his fitness as well.

However, this shift from short-term to long-term isn't all about goals you set. As a matter of fact, some of the FF people don't even have a goal when it comes to exercise. To some of them, it would be like having a goal of being the best tooth brusher on their block.

Some don't need a goal all the time because it won't motivate them any more than they already are. Being fit and healthy is enough of a motivator for them. Mark (FF 30) says, "I just tell myself I want to stay in shape, and it is as simple as that." Whether setting goals will work to help you to become ForeverFit or not, you won't know until you use them. If you are going to set goals, it is best to know how to set and use them to get the most out of them. Steven Chandler, author of *100 Ways to Motivate Yourself* said, "It's not what a goal *is* that matters; it's what a goal *does*." Make sure your goal helps you "do." Letter "I" below will help you do so.

The following is your five-step goal setting session. Remember that many short-term goals added together equal a long-term goal. Henry Ford proved with his assembly lines that any job could be done if one was willing to break it down into small pieces.

Goal Setting Strategies

1. Make sure your goals are F.I.T. **F**=For you, **I**=Inspirational, **T**=Time. "For you" simply means having a goal that is *specific* to *your* desires, not someone else's. If there is a certain weight you want to be, state your goal as "My goal is to weigh X pounds," rather than saying "I want to be my ideal weight." The latter is too general. "For you" also means having a goal that will challenge you, yet is attainable. Break it down into bite-sized pieces that you can handle (see 3 below) Inspirational means that your goal aligns with your life values (see 5 below). You need to have a goal that will get you out of bed on those days you'd rather sleep in. Be sure your Inspirational goal is something you are moving *toward,* as this tends to be more joy-based than moving away from something. Yet another reason to become your ideal weight rather than trying to lose weight. Inspirational is your "so that," which is something that gets deep into your soul. This could be something as simple as "so that I can be a good role model for my children." Time means to be sure to

have a specific deadline for your goal. An example would be "I will be exercising four times per week for one hour consistently by (specific date)."

2. Using the F.I.T. model, develop a long-range mega goal. This can be something that you would dream to be (i.e., being ForeverFit). Setting this goal first can help you create your short-term goals.

3. Set short-term goals that, when added up, will reach your long-range mega goal. The long-term goal can look overwhelming until you break it down into segments. A perfect example is when I have helped clients run long races such as half marathons. Thinking about running thirteen miles seems impossible if you aren't running much at all until you break it down to starting at two to three miles for your long run of the week, and adding merely a half mile a week for three to four months. The task then seems less daunting. You can then break down your short-term goals into shorter-term goals, if needed.

4. Read your goals daily. Out of sight, out of mind. Your goals must remain in front of you often to keep them prioritized.

5. When thinking about whether or not a goal inspires you, see that it lines up with your core life values. See how many of the core life values listed below are important to you:

Acceptance
Attractiveness
Confidence
Courage
Creativity
Discipline
Excitement/passion
Financial stability
Freedom

Fun
Health
Honesty
Integrity
Living on purpose
Peace of mind
Personal growth
Relationships
Respect
Spiritual connection

If you do this activity and your ForeverFit goal doesn't seem to align with your top core values, I would ask you to take a good look at your perspective. For instance, if relationships are an important value and you think your goal of becoming ForeverFit would take away from your relationships, think again. Becoming more fit and healthy will only add to your relationships by making you more confident and at ease around those you care about. As a matter of fact, virtually all of the core values listed are aligned with becoming ForeverFit if you see it from a ForeverFit person's perspective. Go back to the list to see how becoming ForeverFit can enhance every aspect of your core values if you truly look for it. This could be a huge key for your long-term motivation.

Long-term perspectives
The following are a few areas where you can look at the long-term perspective and see how this shift will help you make better decisions in becoming ForeverFit.

1. Weight loss/weight gain
I could go through the math of calories in verses calories out (which, by the way, is only one piece of the "ideal weight" puzzle), but instead I will just ask one question: How long does it take to typically put on weight? If it doesn't happen in a couple weeks, why should you expect it to come off that fast? Long-term thinkers know that if they

just keep doing the right things with exercise and nutrition, they will get to their ideal weight.

2. Injury and illness

It can happen to anyone. You are going along so well and something happens: a strained muscle, twisted ankle, the flu. The short-term thinkers either get off track and quit, or aren't willing to take the time off they need to let themselves heal or get healthy, yielding longer recovery time. This can eventually lead to them having to stop, getting depressed about it, and then quitting all together.

The long-term thinkers realize the quicker they do what they need to do to heal the injury and get healthy, the quicker they can get back to exercise. They realize that this week off doesn't mean anything in the long run. Their whole focus becomes getting better. They will also figure out a way to work around their injuries, if possible. Cathy (FF 5), an avid runner, had surgery on her foot. During this time, we trained her arms and core while her foot healed, and then added in functional training for her legs when her foot was cleared for exercise.

As a matter of fact, recently I got some type of bug that had me feeling a little run down, like I was on the edge of something. Sticking to my own advice, I took the whole week off of exercising, knowing in the long run I would get healthier quicker, which I did. It also never manifested into anything, which it might have had I exercised too hard. By the end of the week, I was back at it and felt so good to be moving my body again. One thing you will hear from ForeverFit people when they are taking time off for illness or injury is how they can't wait to get going again—a great attitude to have when you are out of commission physically.

3. The challenge of the workout

The short-term thinker only thinks about how hard the workout is. The long-term thinkers enjoy the workout because they focus on what the workout is accomplishing for their long-term physical and mental health. An hour of exercise seems like a bargain for the other twenty-three hours in the day that it helps, including sleep.

4. Disease prevention

Diseases are prevented by taking proper action in the short run, but are truly prevented when adding up what you do in the short run over many years.

5. Changing or improving

Shifting to more long-term thinking will also help in the area of changing or improving. Sometimes looking at all of the things you feel you need to improve can seem so overwhelming that you either don't know where to start, or you feel paralyzed and don't even want to begin.

If you begin to feel this way when beginning to add your Morning Meeting or an exercise routine, remember this very important question: "If I just change one major thing each year for the next five years, how much better will I be five, ten, twenty years from now?" Looking at it in this light will help you see that it isn't about changing everything today, but instead it is about where you will be five, ten, twenty plus years from now if you continue to strive for improvement. As you go through your day, keep this question in mind as well as another on a more short-term scale, "If I keep doing what I have been doing today (or this week or this month), where will I be in five years from now?" This is a great way to use the short term to help you out in the long run. You may go out even further and ask, "If I continue to do for the next five years what I have done for the last five years, where will I be compared to making one small improvement at a time?" The only way to change your future is to change your patterns, one at a time. These questions are very powerful ways to begin this shift.

Dr. James Prochaska, in his study of over sixty thousand people in their first month of New Year's resolutions, found that after one month, 45 percent had quit. Did that number seem a bit low to you? It did to me as well. In fact, almost everyone I asked thought it would be more like 90 percent. No wonder so many people fail at their New Year's resolutions or any healthy habit change. They go into their resolution to get in shape thinking they have no chance. I believe a big reason why so many quit within the first month could be because they do not go into exercise looking at it in the long run. They want the quick fix, and if it doesn't happen in the first few weeks, they think it isn't worth the effort. Think about the next five years and how you will feel if you are still exercising.

Shifting from Short Term to Long Term

1. Begin to ask yourself, "What are the long-term effects on my health due to my daily actions?"
2. Understand short-term pain for long-term gain when it comes to exercise.
3. Take the long-term perspectives on exercise mentioned in this chapter and watch your reactions to situations and setbacks begin to change.
4. Remember how your ForeverFit goal aligns with your core values.

CHAPTER 11

There Is No "The Way"

"Our human mind always likes different approaches. There
is richness in the fact that there are so many different
presentations of the way."
The Dalai Lama

This quote from the Dalai Lama refers to the different world religions. He believes that if we would begin to look at what they have in common instead of fighting over their differences, the world would be in an entirely different place. This coming from a man whose true religion is kindness. When looking for your way to become ForeverFit, use the same idea. As you begin to educate yourself more and more and receive different ways of how to exercise, begin to look at their commonalities instead of getting confused because of their differences. Ask yourself what you can use from every new form of exercise and use it. See if it seems like something you can use long-term to enhance your fitness lifestyle and keep that much needed variety your body craves.

Observing all of the different ways people get and stay in shape, I have come to realize there truly is no "the way" to exercise perfectly. This, of course, is exactly the opposite of what most of the infomercials tell you. They attempt to make you feel that their product is "the way" to tone abs, butt, and thighs, and that it will give you the hard bodies found in their commercials if you simply use their product.

I stressed earlier in this book the importance of taking advice from those who have what you want. This said, be sure to be open to the fact that what worked for one person to become ForeverFit or their ideal weight may not work for you. You may have a different mentality when it comes to certain modes of exercise and, therefore, may need a different approach. I'm not saying not to use something that a friend or family member has used successfully. Instead, have your mind open to other possibilities as you are doing your current routine.

The value of variety

Most people crave variety, yet are creatures of habit and are often unwilling to try something new. What is the worst thing that will happen if you try something new, as long as it is safe? You may not like it. Is that such a big risk? This is, however, a good area to talk to a fitness professional about. If you are thinking about trying something new, but aren't sure if it is something that would be safe or good for you to do because of your fitness level or other physical limitations, ask a qualified fitness professional. He or she should be able to guide you in the right direction as to the safety and effectiveness of a new mode of exercise. I still do exercises I did fifteen to twenty years ago. I just keep learning and adding things to vary my routines. This can really help with keeping things interesting and challenging.

Some of the products sold in infomercials are decent enough to add variety and will help to yield good results. Just understand that they may not give you everything you are looking for. The body craves change and needs different stimuli for it to be forced to adapt, which is one big thing you will get out of keeping a variety of exercise options. Keep your body guessing. Just because you see a runner who is skinny, don't think, "If I run, I will look like that." You don't know their genetic makeup, what they are eating, if they strength train, how long they have been running, how many miles per week they put in. Many FF people eventually develop a balanced routine, including strength training to keep lean muscle tissue, yoga or flexibility work, and a variety of cardiovascular exercises. Some get stuck in a rut of doing the same old routines, but no matter what, they keep going.

Does this mean you need to incorporate all of these things into your exercise routine? It depends on a lot of factors. What results do you desire? What types of facilities and equipment do you have access to? But most of all, what will you *do* long term? Don't be afraid to try new things. The fitness industry is constantly coming up with new ways to exercise. Try anything that sparks your interest. Try them long enough to see if you will enjoy them and see if they are getting you the results you desire. If they are, keep them.

Never think you have figured out the perfect combination. Keep switching things up. As the Dalai Lama says, "Our human minds like different approaches." This is kind of like saying variety is the spice of life. Getting bored with what you are doing? Try something you never thought you would. You may not only discover a new form of exercise you may enjoy, but you may also take your fitness to a whole new level. This happened to me when I tried yoga for the first time. I thought I was just going to get a nice stretch and ended up getting not only a good stretch, but also a great workout for my mind, body, and spirit. And I was only taking the beginner class. This also happened to my ForeverFit friend Karyn (FF 11). She took up yoga and at first didn't want to stick with it because she wasn't very good at it. However, she chose to take the perspective that because she wasn't good at it, yoga was a challenge her body needed so she stuck with it, and guess what? She now loves it, is better at it, and now has a new mode of exercise to challenge herself with and keep that much needed variety.

What to ask when trying something new

Be cautious of anyone who says his or her way is the only way to exercise. Don't automatically shrug them off, but at the same time, don't just buy into it. Be smart and do your homework. Ask others who have worked with them. How was their experience? Do you have the same goals as them? Ask opinions of other experts (that aren't going to just try to sell you their idea). Good questions to ask are:

1. Does it have any scientific rationale, and has anyone used it to be successful?
2. Does it sound fun?
3. Does it make sense to me?
4. Can I do it long term?
5. Is it safe?

6. Is it different from what I am currently doing?
7. Do I trust the person who is teaching it to me?

If you answered "no" to any of these questions you may want to get more information before starting it. Be smart and ask questions. Be open enough to at least investigate it.

Thinking that your way is the only way to exercise can keep you in a rut, which yields you exactly the results you are getting. If you like the results you are getting and aren't bored, keep on rocking. When your results begin to stagnate or when you begin to get bored, it is time to shake things up.

John's story

John (FF 25) came to me a disheartened, ForeverFit fifty-something. John had strength trained most of his adult life and had eaten well, had the body of a twenty-year-old, yet was frustrated. Why? It started with a shoulder problem, and then his neck and low back, and then his golf game began to suffer. John wasn't bored. Instead, he was stuck in a rut of doing the same old routine time after time, and his joints were beginning to suffer as a result. He was doing very little functional training to keep stability and flexibility in his muscles and joints; doing the same exercises year after year had worn them down. Like rotating the tires in your vehicles, your exercises need to be rotated around. John was in need of a workout makeover, so that is what we did.

John's neck and low back began to feel much better, his flexibility increased, and he enjoyed the challenges these new routines provided. Good thing he was open to there being another way to exercise. John is a great example of one who has become ForeverFit, but just needed some guidance. It goes to show that no matter how fit you are, it is always good to have an expert there to guide you.

Changing ways

The way for you can, and should, be in constant change. Find a foundation of principles you can stick to long-term and shift around within these principles. For example, if you know that strength training, cardiovascular training, and flexibility work are the three areas you wish to work on, you can choose which ways you want to strength train (whether with a personal trainer, on machines, in a group setting or at home, with videos, etc.), what cardiovascular activities you will participate in (as well as the duration and intensity), and how to learn and perform flexibility exercises. There are endless possibilities and combinations. A qualified fitness professional can show you how to organize these activities, but isn't absolutely necessary if you know yourself and are true to your priorities.

No "the way" to change

Just as there is no "the way" to exercise, there is no "the way" to change your habits to become ForeverFit. I must also remind you of the importance of remaining open and being a constant student, no matter how much you learn. Take something from every ForeverFit person you meet and learn from them. The same thing goes for reading this book. The first time through you will find things that are super helpful in becoming ForeverFit, while others will be totally meaningless to you at this point in your journey. Take and use what you need to right now and set aside others. You may need them at another stage along your path.

Everyone comes into this journey with different things they need to work on. Figuring out your own way may take some trial and error, but make sure you keep up your trials consistently. Don't think that just because someone else used the book their way and had great success that it will automatically work that way for you, too (although it might). On that note, it is important that your Morning Meeting truly be your own, not what someone else wants for you. Individualize it according to your own desires of becoming ForeverFit. This is much more empowering than doing it for reasons that someone else laid out for you.

Dr. Ornish, whom I talked about earlier, has another way of looking at making change. In the Fast Company "Change or Die" article he states, "Radical, weeping, comprehensive changes are often easier for people than small, incremental ones." For example, he says that people who make moderate changes in their diets get the worst of both worlds: "They feel deprived and hungry because they aren't eating everything they want, but they aren't making big enough changes to quickly see an improvement in how they feel, or in measurements such as weight, blood pressure, and cholesterol."

This is here to show you that if changing one small thing at a time isn't working for you, you may need to make sweeping, radical changes so you can see and feel the results quicker. However, if you follow the other concepts in this book, like truly looking long-term and doing it for a more internal reason than external, the numbers won't matter as much for you. Everyone is motivated a little differently so I want you to have the options and the reasons why.

Look at other life successes

Another way of making this book work for you is to look at how you have had success in any other area in your life. If you are successful at work because you keep a schedule, have deadlines and written goals, it would be a good idea to schedule your exercise sessions and have written fitness goals with deadlines. If you have become successful in another area of your life because of a passion for what you do, develop a passion for exercise by focusing on any joy you can find, and build from there. If you have great relationships with family or friends, use whatever is making that part of your life successful and transfer it to becoming ForeverFit. If these are the ways you more naturally have become successful at something else in your life, they will most likely be the better path for you to achieve your fitness goals. If you feel you have never succeeded at anything (which is untrue due to the fact that you are reading these words) then doing *anything* will help.

There is no "the way" fitness examples

The following is a list of some questions about exercise I have been asked over the years that there is not a "the way" answer to. I will explain why this is, as well as offer a common sense approach to them.

1. **What time of day is it best to exercise?** I covered this before. Just remember to exercise at the earliest part of your day when you have the most energy since exercise is about energy output. The bottom line is that you get it in. The later in your day you schedule your workout, the greater the chance of something getting in the way.

2. **Is it better to do cardio before or after strength training?** Try it both ways for a few weeks and see which ones make your strength training feel better, since this requires maximal effort. If you have a short-term goal of running a 5k, on the days you run, you may want to run first, to give it the focus it needs.

3. **Machines or free weights?** All weights are safe if you learn to do them properly. I am not an advocate of machines, but am not totally against them either. The more movements you do that require you to control the movement—exercises with free weights, for example—the better, simply because that is how your body has to work outside of the gym. However, don't totally avoid machines if that is all you have to use. Just try to incorporate both. Also remember the rotating your tires idea from John's story. Machines usually force you into a certain movement pattern, whereas free weights do not, especially if you are switching up the movements you are doing with them. Keep this in mind to keep your muscles and joints more protected. Always remember that any movement, if safe, is better than no movement at all.

4. **High reps or low reps?** If you want what most people do, which is to get leaner, not bigger, stay in a range from ten to twenty reps and you are safe. Shifting the repetitions around in this range will give your body the variety it needs. Intensity is what you want here. Lifting weights doesn't bulk you up, unless you lift super heavy and have enough testosterone in your system to do so, which most of us simply don't.

5. **How long should I cardio train?** Again, variety is the key here. Twenty to sixty minutes is the general range,

unless you are training for an endurance event like a triathlon or marathon, for which you may go past an hour or two in your training. Changing factors such as duration, intensity, and the type of exercise you are doing (walking, running, riding a bike, using an elliptical, swimming, aerobics classes, etc.) is what will benefit you most and give you the most variety.

6. **Should I do a longer, slower walk (low intensity) with a longer duration, or faster (high intensity) and shorter duration?** Your answer here is the same as number five above. Variety is the key, unless you are training for a specific event. As a matter of fact, you burn almost exactly the same amount of calories whether you run a mile or walk a mile. Walking a mile just takes longer to burn the same amount of calories.

ForeverFit people have gotten fit with aerobics tapes, walking, running, personal trainers, books, magazines, working out with a partner, group fitness classes such as yoga, pilates, step aerobics, cardio boxing, strength training, and endless others. It doesn't really matter exactly how they did it, but that they have arrived and are here to stay. Have fun on your way!

Applying "There is no 'the way'"

1. There isn't one magic pill, exercise, or group of exercises. Variety is key.
2. Be willing to try any new way to exercise that is safe and makes sense for you. Only after trying it for a period of time should you decide to keep it as part of your regimen or discard it.
3. Be open to new things and, at the same time, do your research and ask questions.
4. There is no exact "way" to apply ForeverFitU. People with different personalities and different needs will use certain parts at certain times.

CHAPTER 12

We All Have Unmotivated Times

"Patience and perseverance have a magical effect before which
difficulties disappear and obstacles vanish."
John Quincy Adams

Sometimes you just have to suck it up and do it anyway. This chapter is perhaps the most important to learn from, because you *will* have unmotivated times to come. Don't think the FF group is this super motivated group 100 percent of the time. We all get tired. We all have times of stagnation and boredom. We all have times when we just don't want to go to the gym. We're too sore, too busy; we just don't want to put in the effort sometimes. But we still do. Why? The bottom line is we know it is good for us, and we love how we feel when we go anyway, especially during times we really don't want to. As a matter of fact, when I asked the ForeverFit people what they tell themselves on the days when they don't want to exercise, over 90 percent said something to the effect of, *"I know I will feel better when I am done."* I am in *total* agreement with them. This little phrase may be the thing that will get you over every obstacle that comes your way; especially on those days when exercise is the last thing you want to do.

I have had some of my clients use a little notebook entitled "How do I feel?" In this notebook I have my client write down before and immediately after each workout how he or she feels on a one to ten scale. I also encourage having them write down how they feel a few hours later. This helps show them the benefits of how exercise makes them feel, so they can look at it later on days when they feel like a one or two and see how exercise helped raise their internal feelings. Start paying attention to how much better you feel after a workout than before. This awareness can help you immensely.

What unmotivated times may be telling you

Unmotivated times are not a sign of failure. Instead, they are either a sign that you are bored and in need of a workout makeover, or have been over-training and could use a day or two of active rest; that is if you have been working out consistently. If you haven't been working out consistently and are unmotivated, it may be time for a refresher course on some concepts in this book.

I love what fifty-six-year-old Rosie (FF 19) said about boredom: "I work too hard to get bored. I feel those who get bored aren't working hard enough." I have never felt bored when I was having my butt kicked by a good workout. When you feel unmotivated, it may be time to change some of the things you are doing in your Morning Meeting (that is, if you are still having them). If you aren't, that is the first thing to get back into your life. When you go back into *ForeverFitU*, you may be amazed how different parts of it will apply to you more than they did before.

Taking a day or two of active rest is a great time to go on a walk, play with your kids, or play a sport you enjoy like tennis or golf for your physical activity instead of going to the gym. This can help to recharge your batteries and get you excited about how exercise has enabled you to do the things you love much more easily. Mary (FF 27) loves the fact that at age fifty-seven she can do activities with her grown, active children like cross-country skiing.

Some FF people simply say they give themselves a break on days when they are unmotivated. John (FF 25) says, "Sometimes I just need a break. A change of pace is good. Sometimes a four-day break is good, and *then I am ready to get back at it.*" Remember, however, these folks are already ForeverFit. Therefore, if you aren't ForeverFit yet, taking four days off may not be the greatest idea. Notice how John said he is ready to get back at it after his rest. If you aren't ready to get back at it, the rest isn't what you needed.

If you take this active rest break, set a date to go back, (usually less than a week) and stick to it. Schedule it. If you take much longer, it can start to seem too normal to not do your workouts. The next thing you know, even active rest starts to seem like too much work, and you are on the road to sedentary living once again. I am not trying to scare you, but unless you have been exercising for years, it can happen that quickly.

This too shall pass

Just keep reminding yourself during these unmotivated periods that they are temporary and that *everyone* goes through them, even ForeverFit folks. Motivation will return. We all go through it. This too shall pass. Getting through these times and still exercising will prove to you that it is truly temporary. It is part of the development of your understanding the value of exercise in your life. Every time you get through an unmotivated streak and exercise the entire time anyway, you will get a little stronger and a little better at it. Your unmotivated times will become increasingly fewer and shorter as well. Don't get depressed when you are unmotivated. Be excited about getting to the other side. The only way to the other side of this unmotivated time is to go through it. Ask yourself the question, "What can I do today to make my workouts more exciting?" or "What things can I do or say today to get myself more motivated?" Reading the same desires and goals for too long can eventually become just words rather than something that is more meaningful. Many times this non-motivation begins from your wanting to sleep that extra ten to twenty minutes rather than have your Morning Meeting with yourself. If you begin to feel this way, recheck your priorities.

No unmotivated timetable

I cannot predict for you how long an unmotivated time will last, mainly because I do not want you to say, "I have 'x' days left until I am motivated again." I will tell you that the more work you do on some of the concepts in *ForeverFitU,* and the more you listen to the advice of the FF people, the quicker you will get motivated again. Remember some of the stories like Susan's that inspired you. Have your Morning Meeting twice per day if you have to. Most of all—take action. Do it anyway. Your mind and body will thank you. Draw on all of the positive experiences in your past from working out, and motivation will soon return. Since there is no finish line, quitting is not an option.

All FF people have unmotivated streaks. However, none of them ever mentions wanting to quit. Instead they talk about how they will feel when they are done with this non-motivated time; they take the day off and don't worry about it, or they play little mind tricks like saying, "You can take tomorrow off. Just go today." None of the ForeverFit folks I interviewed said they don't ever have these times. They all do.

Applying unmotivated times to your ForeverFit goal

1. Knowing that even ForeverFit people have unmotivated times can help you feel it is okay to feel unmotivated from time to time. It won't last forever.

2. Go anyway. These are the workouts that truly count. Anyone can exercise when they feel good.

3. Become aware of how much better you feel after a workout than you did before it, especially during unmotivated times. Use these times when you go anyway to draw motivation for the next time you don't feel like exercising.

4. If you are bored, switch things up by taking a class or playing a sport you haven't played in awhile.

CHAPTER 13

The Bottom Line

"Happiness is when what you say, what you
think, and what you do are in harmony."
Mohandas Gandhi

"There is no way to happiness. Happiness is the way."
Wayne Dyer

From here on out you have choices to make: whether to believe that becoming ForeverFit can happen for you or not, whether to begin an exercise routine or not, whether to begin to apply what you have read or not, whether to go back and read it all again or not. Regardless of what you choose to do, there is one thing you must do: *find a way to be happy with the choices you make day-to-day.* So often I hear people say how it isn't fair they have to exercise so hard, don't get to eat what they want whenever they want anymore, and, if they do, they gain weight. Do you see how much unhappiness there is in a statement such as that? Not only are they unhappy they are having to workout and eat right, but if they eat cheat foods or skip a workout, they are unhappy as well. Why not be happy you can exercise and that you are doing something healthy for yourself by putting nutritious food into your body? If you miss a workout, find a way to be happy doing whatever else it is you are doing. If you are going to eat ice cream, chocolate, or whatever your cheat food may be, why not *enjoy* it? Don't eat it and at the same time have this feeling of guilt come over you. This takes a pleasurable experience and makes it not so pleasurable by multiplying the not-so-healthy food with the negative emotion of guilt. If you cannot escape the feeling of guilt, then I suggest not having those foods in your house. They are obviously causing more long-term pain than joy, both physically and mentally. We all would rather have more joy than pain in our lives. We have this illusion that certain foods give us joy when in reality this joy may last five to ten seconds and is attached with hours, if not days, of guilt and regret, as well as the physical and mental burden of the inches onto our thighs and waists. Sound like a good exchange?

Cheat foods

Although this book is about making exercise a permanent habit, I have to say something about cheat foods. Be sure to include one or two cheat meals or an entire cheat day into your nutritional regimen per week (that is, unless you have met with a nutrition coach that says otherwise for now). This can help keep you on track in your nutrition the rest of the week when you know you have a cheat meal coming. The spike in calories on your cheat day will actually help rev up your metabolism.

Be sure to eat cheat foods consciously. When you become unconscious that you are eating it, you lose the true enjoyment of it. Savor every bite and guess what? You won't need nearly as much of it to satisfy you. Planning when you cheat shows you are controlling the food rather than it controlling you. If you don't want to do a whole cheat day, plan a couple cheat meals throughout the week.

The mind needs cheat food just like it needs healthy food, just not as much as you may think. Thinking you need a cheat food or dessert every day is just a belief you are carrying with you. Change this to having a dessert every so many days, and eventually this will become your belief. If cheating once in awhile always sends you on a road to Ben & Jerryville, you may need to get rid of some things permanently. Plan your cheats and see if this works for you.

Remember, I am not a nutritionist, but simply giving you ideas of what works for me and has worked for many others. Use these ideas how you wish.

Seek overall wellness and balance

Start the enjoyment process by refocusing on what makes you truly, more permanently happy—having a feeling of wellness. This comes from moving your body, putting healthy food into it, keeping your attitude in check, and having a good sense of your spiritual nature. Cheat once in awhile, take a day off once in awhile, and enjoy that too. The body needs rest like it needs to move. Work and rest need to remain in balance. Just make sure your rest is something you truly enjoy.

No more beating yourself up for a bad day or week. Start each day as another chance to see yourself back at the gym. Each day is a day to meet with yourself and ask, "What can I improve upon today?" Wayne Dyer said, "True nobility is not being better than someone else, but being better than I used to be." Begin to ask yourself, "What can I do today to be better than I used to be," and at the end of the day, ask, "In what ways was I better today than I used to be?" Do it with a right attitude and with happiness. Bring happiness to all of your endeavors, success will chase you, and you will be ForeverFit before you know it and will enjoy the process a whole lot more!

Applying the bottom line to your ForeverFit goal

1. Be happy with the choices you make day to day.
2. Enjoy your cheat foods, just not as often.
3. Seek overall wellness and balance in your life.

Chapter 14

Paying it Forward

**"As a parent, it is my job to live my life the way I would one
day like my children to live theirs."**
Scott Fjelsted

Even if you aren't a parent yet, read this section. You may have nieces, nephews, brothers, sisters, cousins, and friends whose habits are being influenced by yours. You are constantly influencing those around you whether you know it or not. If you can't become ForeverFit for yourself, do it for the next generation. According to the American Obesity Association we live in a country where currently 30 percent of children are overweight and 15 percent are obese. This is a 400 percent rise in overweight and obese children from 1975 to 2000, and it is only getting worse, due to more and more sedentary living and overeating. Children with at least one obese parent are almost twice as likely to be overweight as children with normal weight parents. The problems from this excessive weight are endless and include diabetes, heart disease (yes, even in young adults), high blood pressure, bone and joint problems, sleep apnea, as well as the psychological and social issues of being an overweight child.

Monkey see, monkey do

While genetics always play at least a little role in anything, really take a look at the habits you are passing along to your children. I learned with my two boys that if I told them to do something but wasn't doing it myself, they weren't doing it either. This revelation came to me when I began to do the "What do you say?" routine when someone gave them something. What I didn't realize is how little they heard the words *thank you* come out of *my* mouth. As I expressed gratitude more to others in front of them, their thank you behavior improved. Watch the actions you take (or don't take) on a daily basis, especially when it comes to activity and eating. Get rid of the "Do as I say, not as I do" routine.

A mother's FF influence

I owe so much of becoming ForeverFit to my mother. She showed me, by her actions, not her words, that exercise can be a normal part of life. Every day she would be up between four and five in the morning doing her exercise routine. These were the days before exercise mats so she actually wore an area down in the carpet from all of her dancing around. My room was downstairs, and I remember knowing it was time for me to get up when I heard her get into a certain part of her routine. The floor would creek a certain way and it became my alarm clock. She would then walk over two miles to work. After work, she would walk home, make us dinner, and then go on a walk with neighbor friends. We never thought she was compulsive or exercised too much, and never heard her talk about it or complain that she had to do it. It was just an expected part of her day. I thank her so much for what she was showing me, not by lecturing, but by her daily actions.

It is never too late!

Even if your children are grown and you have never exercised a day in your life, you can now show them it is possible to become ForeverFit at any age, and can be a source of inspiration to them. If you are a parent of younger children as I am, you have an amazing opportunity in your hands. Use your children to inspire you to become ForeverFit, thereby helping them to become ForeverFit in their own lives without the struggles so many have to go through. My mother proved that if you are ForeverFit, your children can be, too.

It is our obligation as parents to be an example to our children. It is our obligation to show them how we truly put what is most important in life first. When we feel like we don't want to take time away from our children to exercise, we need to understand what values we are showing them by exercising—that our health is important to us and that we will be so much happier when we are done exercising. We will become better parents after exercising, and we will have more energy to play with them. But, most of all, they will see us doing our exercises and one day they will ask to join us. I actually saw the daughter of Tina (FF 25) in a group bike class at 5:30 in the morning—without Tina. And she is only a sophomore in high school. Tina has given such a great gift to her daughter by showing her the value of a healthy lifestyle, and her daughter is already beginning her ForeverFit journey at sixteen.

Exercise as a family

If you still can't see yourself taking time away from the family to exercise, how about exercising as a family? When you exercise as a family, you get to enjoy family bonding while you get fit, as well as show your family how much fun fitness can be. Whether it be getting a Wii Fit and having an active game night to playing sports with your family and others in your neighborhood to simply going on walks or bike rides, make it something all can participate in. Keeping the environment fun is key. Competitiveness is fine as long as fun is the underlying theme. Hop on the web and look for other ideas you can do together as a family.

My wife and I walk the family dog, Ellie Mae, with the boys most nights after work, even in the wintertime. This can last anywhere from thirty minutes to over an hour, depending on how much we play. It is a great natural way, outside of their normal playtime, that we can spend quality time together in nature and get physical activity in at the same time. We sometimes play "tag," which throws in some good interval training as we chase each other. In the winter, we slide down a hillside in our snow pants. Climbing the hill adds great variety to our walk. We also like to play the Wii in the winter and go swimming in the summer. Little things like this can carry over to their adult lives. I am so blessed to have a wife that enjoys physical activity as much as I do. If your spouse is not interested in joining you yet, you can find another family member or close friend to exercise with until your spouse does decide to join you.

Inspiring others by becoming ForeverFit

This obligation to pay it forward is not a guilt thing. It is meant to be inspirational. Every person who becomes more active shows many others how great exercise is for them. Every time you feel healthier, look better, have more energy, get closer to your ideal weight, you may only help one other person to get on the road, but that is one more person that is on the fitness track that wouldn't have been if it weren't for you. This person then has the opportunity to do exactly what you did for them for someone else, and the snowball effect has begun. Do you see the importance here? Don't nag others to exercise. Be an example and keep talking about how great you feel. They will wonder what you are doing and want to get on board. If you can't seem to motivate yourself, get your mind off of yourself and decide you will become an inspiration to others by becoming ForeverFit.

When I asked my ForeverFit friends and family members, "How long did it take for exercise to feel like a normal part of life?" the ones who began exercising in their teenage years virtually all answered "right away." It is a whole lot easier to establish these healthy habits at a younger age before you have all of the other things going on such as careers, spouses, kids, etc. I am sure Tina's daughter would agree.

ForeverFit as your purpose

So many are searching for a purpose in life. Unfortunately in our society, most feel this is in the form of some type of career when in reality it often simply comes down to helping humanity in one way or another, whether it is our children or a stranger. Maybe your outward purpose at this moment in your life is to show others that becoming ForeverFit is possible regardless of your age, weight, sex, upbringing, financial situation, physical limitations, current career situation, or anything else. Maybe you are someone who never thought you could become ForeverFit, but now are developing a knowing that you can, and one day will be. The more others think you can't do it makes the story all the better when you do. Let this become your outward purpose for now, to show your children and others that becoming ForeverFit is a matter of choice, not chance.

Imagine what this generation of overweight and obese children face. They are going to one day have children of their own, and if the cycle isn't interrupted, they are going to raise more unhealthy kids. Education is part of the battle, but it all starts with what they see on a daily basis. Something has to balance out the onslaught of fast food and soda pop commercials, and the social acceptance of being sedentary and overweight. This is the most socially acceptable epidemic there has ever been, and something needs to be done to make us a healthier world. Begin by becoming ForeverFit yourself.

Applying paying it forward to your ForeverFit goal

1. Remember that children will follow more of what you do than what you say.
2. Exercise as a family.
3. If you don't have a sense of purpose, make becoming ForeverFit your purpose for now to inspire others to do the same.

CHAPTER 15

Conclusion

I have covered a lot of strategies in this book to help you become ForeverFit, including having your Morning Meeting, watching your attitude, gaining perspective, reprioritizing, focusing on the joys of exercise, asking proper questions, and creating the right pictures in your mind. For the last time, repetition is the key not only to learning, but also to making new habits relatively unconscious acts. Throughout, I have laid out simple ways to begin this process and tasks to do during your Morning Meeting. Take from this what you will and do it your way. Just begin by doing something, anything. Beginning is actually much easier than thinking about beginning. Talk to a trainer. Find a good book on exercise. Talk to someone who is ForeverFit and ask him or her what he or she does. Ask him or her to be your accountability partner. Read portions of this book again. Go on a walk. Join a gym. Get a workout partner. As Albert Einstein said, "Nothing happens until something moves." Keep making steps forward. Don't worry about the steps back. They are part of the process. Remember, it isn't about being perfect, but about being better than you used to be.

The following is something I stumbled upon that I wrote months before I began writing *ForeverFitU*. I wrote it in the wee hours of the morning, while listening to the morning breeze. The interesting thing is how well it summarizes the ideas in this book more beautifully than I could now. The first thing to note is how it starts, with a question to myself to which I let my mind search for the answer. It is amazing how clear things appear to you when the world is silent at 3:30 in the morning. Patanjali said, "When you are inspired by an extraordinary project, your consciousness expands in every direction." It is interesting how I wrote this months before the writing of this book began and is being used years later as part of its conclusion. I am just glad I kept it.

Why Exercise?

The ego wants you to sit your butt on the couch, use remote controls, and avoid as much pain as possible. But eventually you come to a conclusion that you can't go on this way—lazily. So you decide to exercise and start eating right. But instead of doing it for deeper reasons like health, vitality, or treating your body like what it was designed for, you instead say, "I want to lose weight or look a certain way." You get focused on external rewards, which, as you know from other things in life, will fade over time. Even if you were to get six-pack abs, if that was your goal, you would then keep working out for the fear of losing them—or in other cases, going back to your old weight, etc.

Basing goals on these externals is uninspiring. It may get you to start but will never keep you going. Joy must rule. Start looking deeper, and you will see that exercise, which is perceived by most as a chore, actually becomes a privilege. For many, it becomes the one time in their day where they can forget about all their worries, get their natural endorphins flowing, increase energy and decrease stress—another huge reason to exercise as early in the day as possible. Why not be able to use this added energy for your day?

We each have our deep, inspiring reason to exercise. A great question to ask is, "If I were to be at a ten in my fitness and nutrition, what would that add to the rest of my life? What things would I like to be able to do that I'm not doing now?" This may open the door to things you haven't thought of in years, or maybe ever. Maybe there is a sport you used to play when you were younger that you would like to get back into. Maybe you have never played a sport and would like to try but have been too out of shape. Maybe there are children or grandchildren in your life or on the way and you not only want to be around for them, but also want to be an active part of their lives. Your desire is to be a good role model and to pass on the legacy of health and wellness to them. The list goes on and on. Bottom line: Your reason has to be individualized and something based on joys instead of fears. Externals are okay, but without the deep, burning desire an internal knowing brings, you are destined for more struggles and, eventually, failure.

Once you have utilized these principles and strategies consistently—long enough to become ForeverFit—you will continue to see all of the benefits they bring. Use this new energy, vitality, and confidence to help you in all of life's endeavors, whether it be in faith, family, work, or play. I am glad you have made it this far in the book. If you are this persistent with becoming ForeverFit, you will be there before you know it. Remember that like life, becoming ForeverFit is more a journey than a destination.

As the ancient Chinese proverb goes: "The best time to plant a tree was twenty years ago. The second-best time is now."

May your Forever begin now!

Now do something, anything, **in a positive direction and** have fun **on your journey!**